The A

Vinegar Bible

Nature's Way For

Weight Loss, Detoxing

Healthy Skin And Ailments Problems

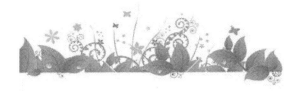

Elena C Hutchinson

Copyright, Legal Notice and Disclaimer

ISBN-13: 978-1492864486

The Apple Cider Vinegar Bible

Nature's Way For Weight Loss

Detoxing, Healthy Skin And

Ailments Problems

Heart Healthy Recipes for Better Health

And A Longer Life!

Elena C Hutchinson

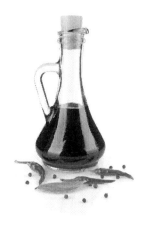

DEAR READER!

✓ What if you could naturally alter your tastes so the foods that you like to eat would be the same foods which make you healthier?

✓ What if you were able to boost your energy, sleep much better, enhance your mood and get rid of weight?

✓ And imagine if you were able to remove the symptoms of your illness - merely by altering the food that you put in your plate?

The Apple-Cider Vinegar Bible is really an essential resource that incorporates cutting-edge advice on vinegar's remarkable health and wellness benefits with a variety of useful home and beauty tips.

Discover the astonishing power of ACV - now recognized as a valuable weight loss and detoxing element. Learn how to make use of vinegar to assist in preventing ailments like bone loss, arthritis as well as cardiovascular disease.

You'll find a broad variety of home treatments (home remedies) for healing psoriasis, eczema, allergies, toothache, sore throat, sunburn, and more. Environmentally friendly household tips and tasty, Heart Healthy Recipes.

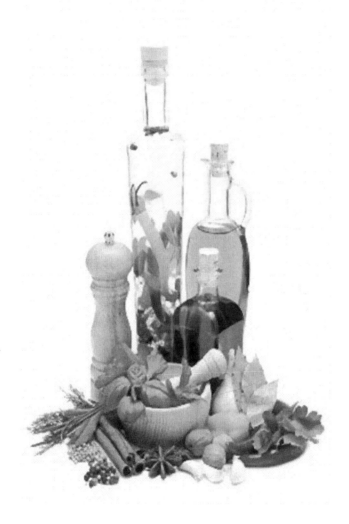

CONTENTS

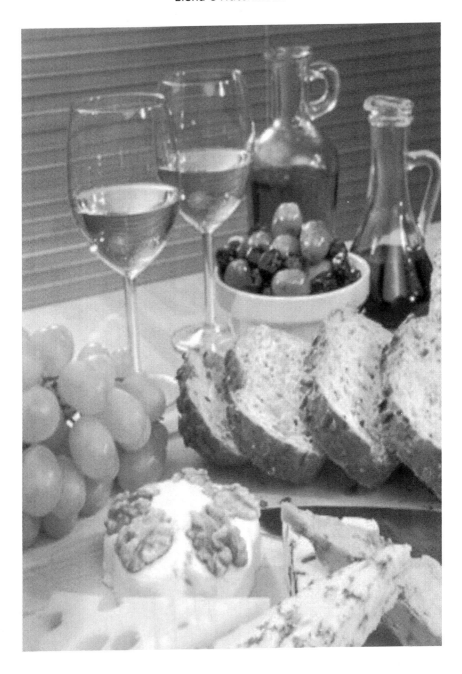

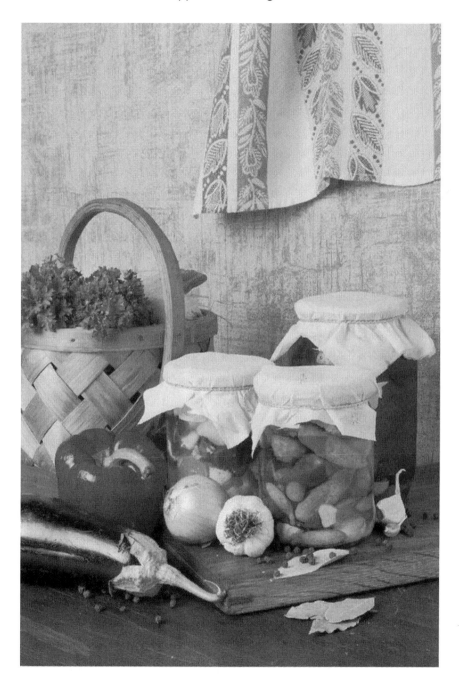

ACKNOWLEDGEMENT

I want to thank my parents for always believing in me no matter what wild ideas I came up with, and my husband Jason, my one and only honey. Also, to our amazing kids, Jane, Gwyneth and Shemar— looks like we knocked it out of the park.

FOREWORD

When I first became familiar with cider vinegar in the seventies, I found it enjoyable. I began to read reports of its effectiveness in the treatment and cure of minor health problems: it appeared to work well in the sort of issues that physicians call chronic, meanings that; they do not know how exactly to treat them.

Even with various case histories of individuals who had found remarkable relief with cider vinegar within their daily conditions, the medical establishment often disregarded the claims of cider vinegar out of hand, as they were not part of a scientifically measured trial.

Clearly, we need more scientific research to back up personal experience; however a broad selection of anecdotal sources would indeed suggest that it works. It's now over sixteen years since I first became interested in cider vinegar; but its use for these conditions can be as frequent as ever.

Whether your interest is really in food which is both healthy and delicious, or in finding out if it works for you personally like a remedy, you can't afford to be without vinegar.

INTRODUCTION

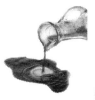

inegar has been produced and used for thousands of years: in fact, vinegar is the only storable food because it can be kept for an almost unlimited period with no expiry date.

The "Father of Medicine', Hippocrates (460-370 BC) is known to have recommended vinegar to his patients in order to renew the four humors into a balanced harmony. They were also the first to flavor vinegar with spices and herbs.

Apple cider vinegar originates from apple cider. The cider is fermented into alcohol, and the alcohol is allowed to continue fermenting until it becomes vinegar. All vinegar is created in this way; if you allowed your wine in your cupboard to continue fermenting, in the course of time, you'd have vinegar.

For centuries, apple cider vinegar is prescribed as a miracle remedy to treat all types of ailments - some cured, some not - and together with the resurgence of naturopathy in recent years, the vinegar has found itself back within the health limelight.

What can this unbelievable vinegar do to help you? In an environment of growing obesity rates, the most prized property of apple-cider vinegar is the way it can suppress appetite.

A recent research found a positive correlation between the amount of vinegar consumed and appetite suppression. Apple cider vinegar is prized for a completely different motive - it's shown to reduce blood sugar.

One study demonstrated that type-2 diabetics (without insulin shots) who took only two tablespoons of vinegar before going to bed were discovered to get far more stable levels of blood sugar each day.

Apple-cider vinegar is an inexpensive; all natural therapy that's virtually sure to enhance your wellbeing, should you endure type-2 diabetes, pre-diabetes or weight - associated insulin resistance, apple-cider vinegar is an inexpensive, all natural treatment that is sure to better your health. Studies also have discovered that vinegar can ease hypertension and lower cholesterol.

It's really not yet known whether these same effects will be seen in human. One study has demonstrated that individuals who consume vinegar based salad dressing at least five times weekly were at a significantly reduced risk of cardiovascular disease.

Further study will probably be necessary to nail the precise connection between cardiovascular disease and apple-cider vinegar; however, these early results are exceptionally promising.

HEALTH BENEFITS OF VINEGAR

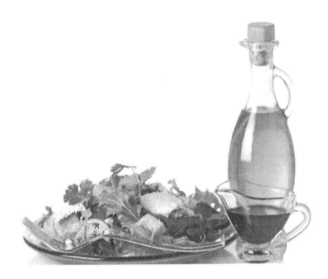

Prior to the developments in modern medicine, vinegar, being accessible to the overall population, was utilized as a curative in many ways. It was- and still is-the foundation for many home remedies.

One could challenge most of the curative remedies credited to vinegar nevertheless vinegar certainly has properties which have helped in many different circumstances.

There are claims that vinegar can reduce osteoporosis, lengthen life, treat arthritis and dementia, and enhance hearing, eyesight and mental powers. There are still lots of ways that vinegar can be healthful both internally and externally, while all this could be well beyond its reasonable qualities.

All of the health benefits linked to vinegar is associated with cider vinegar made from apple cider or a base of processed apple parts. ACV has the same advantages of other vinegars and differs only because it is created from the juice pressed from apples.

Cider vinegar is the most common in America due to the abundance and accessibility of apples. Hard cider (historically a home-made, American alcoholic drink) upsurge to the normal utilization of cider vinegar.

Natural apple-cider that you just see within the health-food store isn't processed in the same manner, and that's the reason you'll generally find sediment in the bottom of these bottles.

VINEGAR IN YOUR SPRAY BOTTLES

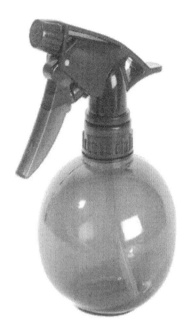

A splash straight from the bottle works just fine in lots of circumstances. Vinegar can work full strength diluted with water or not. Spray bottles are a fantastic way to dispense vinegar full strength.

Whether you reuse small bottles you have cleaned out, or purchase new ones check out travel bottles or spray bottles within the drug store cosmetic area-you may wish to keep spray dispensers of full strength vinegar by every sink.

Within the kitchen you might prefer a larger, colored one on your own counter. Make use of a permanent marker to clearly label "vinegar" on any bottle in which it is kept.

Vinegar in spray bottles is great for spraying the counters or spraying peeled potatoes which is used in potato salad to keep them from discoloring. Make use of a permanent marker to clearly label "vinegar" on any bottle in which it's stored.

VINEGAR IN YOUR FOOD

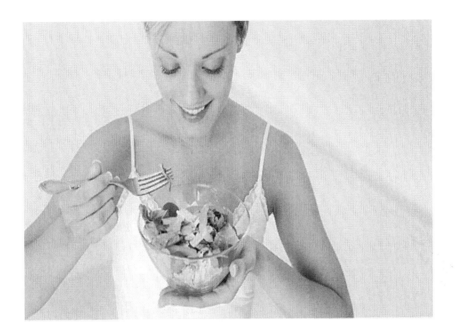

Vinegar is safe and edible, and it cannot hurt your stomach when ingested in small quantities. Multiple sorts and flavors of vinegars are available, in regards to food enhancements and vinaigrettes.

The world of culinary vinegars is a big one. Many types of vinegar are flavored by the addition of herbs or fruits; raspberry vinegar is one of the very popular. For the diet conscious, vinegar is fat free and low in sodium.

TRUSTED HEALTH TREATMENT

A Cleaner, and Neutralizer For Your Kitchen

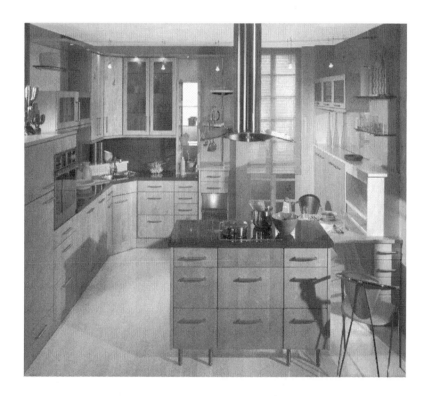

Vinegar has been a kitchen staple for a number of generations. It is really a trusted health treatment, a cleaner, a neutralizer, a condiment along with a preservative. Its acetic value permits it to eliminate germs, mold and bacteria while being secure enough to not harm the body or the environmental surroundings.

50 grains is the same as a 5% acid level, and it is probably the most frequent percent. Since distilled white vinegar isn't registered as a pesticide the label cannot claim it as a disinfectant.

Vinegar is available in higher acetic concentrations; however this is not easy to find in consumer shops as it can be more risky and needs to be handled with suitable precautions.

Use basic white distilled vinegar when a sharp acidity is desired without the other features. Its nutrients are destroyed by the distilling process, making it a purer and much sharper acetic acid and clear in color. Many types of vinegar in stores today also have preservatives added.

Malt vinegars and brown rice vinegars are most frequently used in combination with "fish recipes." Distilled vinegar used for making pickles functions best with at least a 5% or higher acidity level. Always read the label carefully. In case it says wine vinegar, then it is vinegar, not wine.

Asian supermarkets generally carry three basic types of rice vinegar - black, red and white. As rice (the base) features a taste rice vinegars are normally milder.

The popular flavored rice vinegars have a mixture of sweeteners and salt added giving it a light taste. It has turned into a healthy option for all, like a salad dressing plus a flavor enhancer.

Use Vinegar As Your Liquid Cleaner

For cleaning purposes, it is wise to use distilled 5% acid white vinegar. Cider or brown vinegar ought to be avoided for cleansing since it may cause certain surfaces to stain.

No vinegar ought to be utilized on marble surfaces, in metal goblets or on unglazed pottery that may be decorated with leaded paint.

It could leach into the liquid. If you see that straight vinegar or a vinegar and water solution doesn't clean as you had hoped, it could be a result of a slight residue previous commercial cleaners have remaining. If so you will need to add 1/2 teaspoon of detergent to your own water and vinegar solution.

A cleaning solution can vary from 2 parts water to 1 part vinegar or 3 or 4 parts water to 1 part vinegar, depending on the strength you wish to work with. Vinegar is a safe and economical cleaner that may be used in place of several other industrial cleaning supplies.

How To Make Your Very Own Vinegar

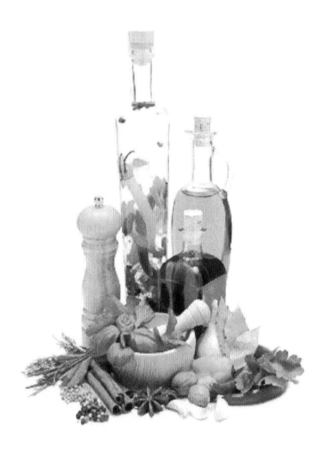

First you begin with a sweet based fluid of your option as it can be created from anything containing sugar or starch. Cider or aged wine or a different fruit juice is usually the simplest to use.

The top of your container should be covered with cheesecloth, but not air tight as you'll need the bacteria in the air to allow it to ferment. It may look bad but it is good. If your vinegar seems too strong, add a little water.

Once you are happy with the flavor, transfer the liquid into a clean bottle through a paper coffee filter. Seal with a cork (the vinegar will corrode a metal top). Keep your vinegar in a dark warm place. This is not a quick process. It will take many weeks to several months - or more - to produce vinegar that you will enjoy.

Fruit Vinegars

The most popular include apple, raspberry, quince, pineapple, coconut and date. Try experimenting with your own fruit wines, using the same procedure as for home-made wine vinegar.

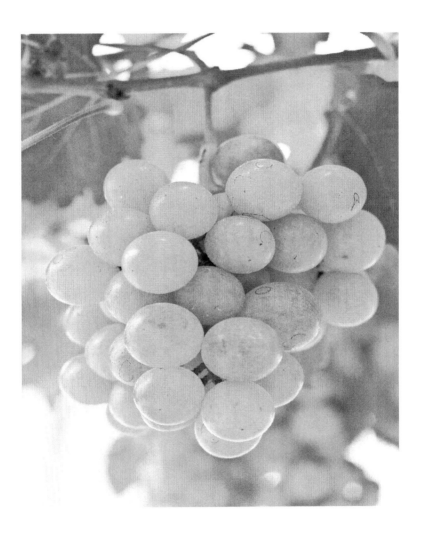

Delicious Vinegar Pie Recipe

This is very delicious and easy to make.

Ingredients:

4 eggs

1-1/2 cups sugar

1 tbsps. vanilla

2 tbsps. vinegar (white, cider, balsamic or rice)

1/4 cup margarine or butter, melted

9-inch frozen pie shell, defrosted

Direction:

Preheat oven to 350°. In big dish mix butter, vanilla, eggs, vinegar, sugar and. Mix well and pour into the defrosted (or homemade) pie shell. Bake 50-60 minutes until firm. Cool. Top, if desired, with whipped cream.

Classic Puddle Cake Recipe

Tasty, and easy to make.

Ingredients:

1 cup sugar

1-1/2 cups flour

1 teaspoon baking soda

4 tablespoons cocoa powder

1 tablespoon vinegar

Make 3 small (holes) in the dry mixture, then insert 1 teaspoon vanilla flavoring or 4 tablespoons cooking oil or 1 tablespoon vinegar in the "hole".

(Choose only one)

Direction:

Pour 1 cup water over the mixture and stir with a fork until evenly blended with the dry ingredients.

Bake at 3500 for 40 minutes.

VINEGAR NUTRITION

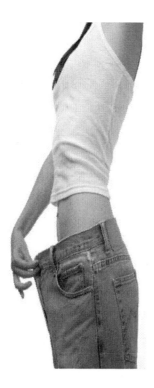

It is often these elements giving vinegar its healthful qualities and nature, although most commercial vinegar these days is filtered to take out the main source "the mother" as well as any sediment.

It's very sad that, lots of people feel vinegar is a superior product as it is more aesthetically appealing, so producers comply by pasteurizing and filtering the vinegar they make. This process stops the activity of the acetobacter bacteria.

The end result is vinegar whose quality may be regulated and assured, but is lacking a number of the critical qualities that makes it so successful for health benefits. Removing the "mother" and sediments of vinegar also lessens the complexity of flavors in the vinegar.

Like processed flour and pasteurized juices which have had nutrients removed or destroyed, vinegar which is filtered and pasteurized could be commercially acceptable, but less successful nutritionally.

Apples are nutritional powerhouses and truly deserving of the legendary phrase; an apple a day keeps the doctor away. They feature a wide variety of nutrients, such as pectin (soluble fiber), beta-carotene (an antioxidant), and lots of minerals.

CHAPTER 1

VINEGAR IN YOUR COOKING

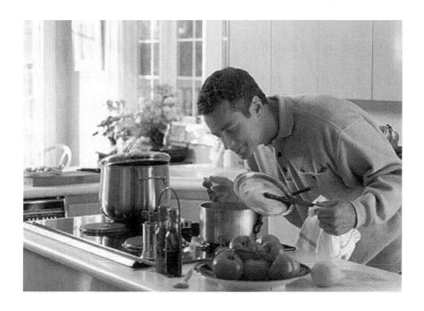

Because vinegar tenderizes meat, it's really a common ingredient in meat marinades. It is always a good addition when slow cooking any tough, cuts of meat. A vinegar and sugar mix is the foundation for an easy sweet - and - sour taste that will be another reason it's found in lots of recipes.

Lemons are offered year-round today, which was not always the case. Vinegar was regularly used as a lemon flavor substitute. The same taste function is performed by its acid base, though vinegar does not possess the Vitamin C value of lemon. Vinegar was and is used as a preservative, particularly crucial before refrigeration. Our fondness for pickling recipes derives from this custom.

Vinegar On Your Meat

- Consider using vinegar to wash virtually any meat, including poultry, to kill bacteria.

- Rub vinegar on the cut end of uncooked ham to prevent mold.

- Add some tablespoons of either cider vinegar or white vinegar to boiling ham to lower the salty taste and make the meat more flavorful.

- Marinate meat in vinegar both to kill bacteria and also to tenderize the meat. A quarter cup of vinegar, added to any other liquid ingredients, is enough for a two- to three-pound roast. Include your favorite herbs to add flavor to the dish. Wine vinegars are great for marinating.

- Add a tablespoon of vinegar when boiling ribs or stew meat for extra tenderness.

Basting And Marinating Your Meat Using Vinegar

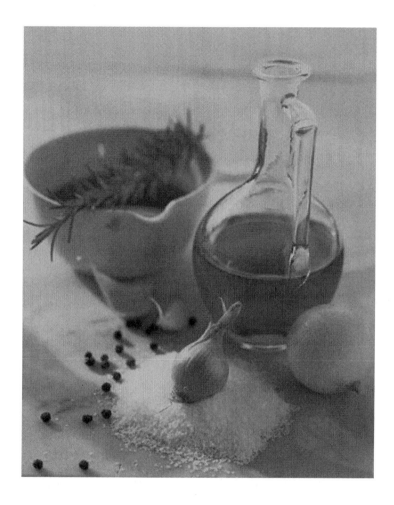

Let less tender meats rest several hours in a glass dish or a durable plastic bag in a marinade before cooking. Steak, for one, gains from this procedure. You too can marinate meat in a zip closing bag and keep it in the freezer until ready to use. Or perhaps a marinade can be utilized only to baste meats as they cook on a grill or in the oven.

Meat Basting Sauce

Mix 1/2 cup sugar (white or brown), 1/4 cup rice vinegar, 1/4 cup ketchup, 2 tablespoons soy sauce, 2 crushed garlic cloves, 1 teaspoon fresh ginger (or 1/4 teaspoon ginger powder) and 2 tablespoons corn-starch. Cook on medium heat until it boils. Stir until it thickens a bit.

Simple Beef Marinades

Mix 1/2 cup white or rice vinegar

1/4 cup oil

1/4 cup

ketchup

1 cup brown sugar and 5 tablespoons soya sauce, or make a quick marinade sauce using equal parts of a prepared barbecue sauce and vinegar. You may need to add more sugar to taste. (This has more of a smoky flavor)

Vinegar On Your Eggs

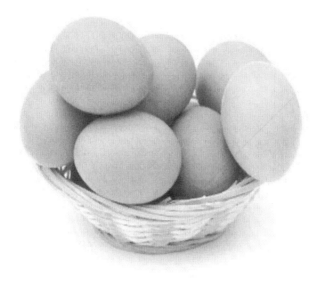

- Replace an egg when baking, in case you are short one egg for a recipe, with a tablespoon of white wine vinegar. This can work only if there is another rising agent present, for example baking soda, baking powder or self-rising flour.

- Add a tablespoon or two of white vinegar to water when boiling eggs to help keep them from cracking and to limit the whites from leaking, in the event the shells split.

- Add a little vinegar to the water when poaching eggs. The whites stay better formed. You can use an empty tuna can (top and bottom removed) for a fast poached egg form.

- Make creamy scrambled eggs. Add a tablespoon of vinegar for every two eggs used, as eggs thicken when scrambling and stir until eggs are done.

Vinegar On Your Fish

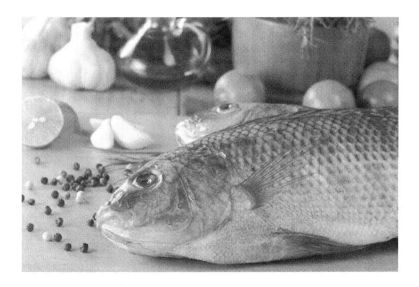

- Try adding a tablespoon of white vinegar to any fish or seafood you are frying or poaching to make it tastier.

- Season fish with a tablespoon of herbal flavored vinegar "for example" tarragon for a different taste.

- Marinate seafood or canned fish ahead, about 20 minutes in vinegar and water to make it taste fresher.

- Rub fish with vinegar a few minutes before scaling, to make the procedure easier.

- Create an enjoyable sauce for serving over hot, cooked fish by combining 2 teaspoons white wine vinegar with 1/2 cup heavy cream.

Vinegar On Your Veggies Tips

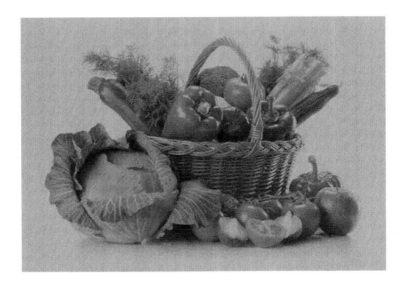

- Eliminate bugs in almost any fresh veggies with a short soak in water using a good dash of salt and vinegar.

- Add one or two spoonful of vinegar and soak them in cold-water to freshen wilted vegetables.

- Top cooked chilled asparagus with any vinaigrette of your desire.

- Store fresh bell peppers in sterilized jars, and top off with boiling vinegar. Seal tightly. Store two weeks before serving.

- Olives and pimentos covered with vinegar will last almost indefinitely if refrigerated.

Using Vinegar To Make

A Creamy Coleslaw Dressing

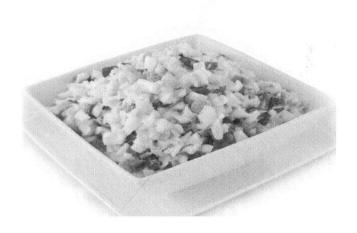

1 tablespoon vegetable oil

2 tablespoons sugar

1/4 cup seasoned rice vinegar

1/2 teaspoon dry mustard

Add salt and pepper to taste

Try Colonel's Coleslaw

Dressing By Combining

1/3 cup sugar

¼ cup milk

¼ cup buttermilk

½ tablespoons white vinegar

½ tablespoons lemon juice

½ cup mayonnaise

Add salt and pepper to taste

Vinegar On Your Fruits

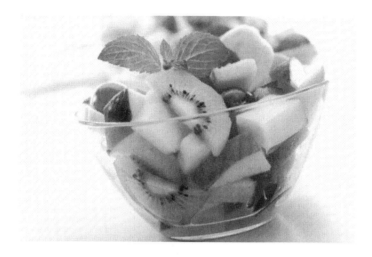

- Enhance the flavor of any fruit you are cooking by including a little vinegar.

- Create a fast fruit dressing by including a couple of tablespoons of the fruit-flavored vinegar with both a cup of sour cream or vanilla yogurt.

- Splash a little rice or balsamic vinegar on fresh fruits for example pears, cantaloupe, honeydew or others to put in a zesty new flavor.

Serve immediately to prevent the fruit from becoming mushy.

Combine and serve.

Vinegar On Your Carbs

- Add a teaspoon of vinegar to the boiling water to get amazing results with your rice.

- Add just a dash of vinegar to pasta since it cooks, to cut some of its own starch and to help it become less starchy.

- Season cold pasta with any vinaigrette. Make it a full meal with the addition of cubes of meat, ham or chicken along with cheese and cooked vegetables for example peas and shredded carrots.

- Keep peeled potatoes from discoloring for short term use (or even for days, in the event you want, by storing them in the fridge), by covering them with cold-water to which some vinegar was added.

- Give homemade bread a shiny crust by brushing the very top of a loaf with vinegar a few minutes before baking is ended. Return to the hot oven to complete.

Pickling With Vinegar

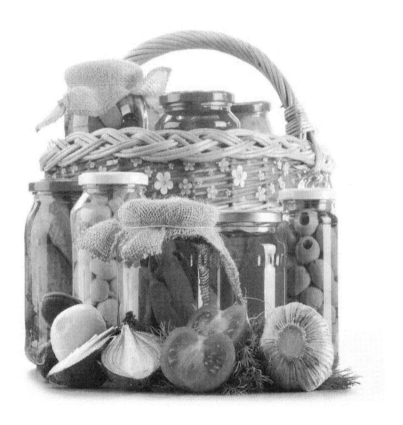

Pickling with vinegar is really a centuries old approach of preserving food. It is used less now for preserving food than for making pickles. Vinegar creates an atmosphere where bacteria cannot live mainly because of the acid content.

This is actually the reason you need to utilize glass or ceramic containers for pickling because the acid will not react with it while it might react to metal and even some plastic pickling containers.

There are three types of vinegar used in setting up pickles. Most recipes call for white distilled vinegar, which has a distinctive odor plus a lemony flavor. It will not alter the color of light veggies or fruits. Apple cider vinegar, frequently used in pickling, has its unique fruity flavor and it may trigger many meals to darken.

It is essential that you follow pickling recipes carefully. Do not use any flavored vinegars, and unless that's particularly called for do not dilute the vinegar with water. Perhaps you'll find some favorites within your household that you should remember to write-down.

Selecting the correct size and type of cucumber is part of the art. Smaller pickle cukes, for instance, make crisper pickles. When making pickles if working in quantity, you can clean a whole load of cukes in your top-loading clothes washer. Just remember to line underneath with a towel, utilize a cold-water wash, gentle cycle, though a dab of vinegar will not hurt.

- Make a big jar of fridge pickles. First place in a big, broad - mouth glass jar, 1 cup of sugar and 1 cup of very hot water. Stir until the sugar dissolves.

Include 1/2 cup of white vinegar and stir again. Now add to the jar thin, circle-sliced pieces of two cucumbers and one bunch of green onion tops cut in J-inch pieces. Cover the bowl and store in the fridge at least a half day before serving.

This Makes an Excellent

Sweet and Sour Pickle

These will keep for just two months in the refrigerator.

Place several small, hard-cooked, peeled eggs in a broad-mouth jar with a small sliced onion.

In a pan, bring to a boil and simmer over low heat for about 5 minutes:

3 cups vinegar

3-inch cinnamons stick

1 tablespoon honey

1 teaspoon each whole spice and whole clove.

1/2 teaspoon whole coriander seeds (optional), a slice of fresh ginger the size of a quarter and a bay leaf.

Once cooled, pour this mixture over the eggs and refrigerate for a week before using.

Vinegar On Your Dairy

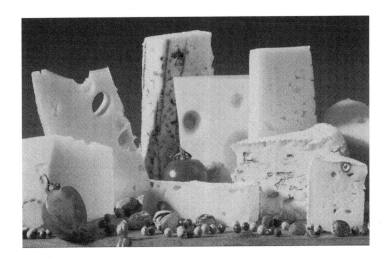

- Keep cheese fresh for longer by wrapping it in a cloth moistened with vinegar. For additional protection, keep the cheese in a sealed container.

- Make a substitute, low-fat sour cream, by blending in a food processor a 12 oz. container of small curd cottage cheese with 1/4 to 1/3 cup. skim milk, 2 teaspoons vinegar, and 2 teaspoons sugar.

- Make a buttermilk substitute by adding a tbsp. of vinegar to a cup of fresh milk and let stand long enough to thicken 5 to 15 minutes. Speed the procedure up by microwaving the mixture for 30 40 seconds.

- Give a little extra zest to your white sauce by adding 1/2 teaspoon of your preferred vinegar.

Vinegar Tips And Ideas

Cider Vinegar And Pork

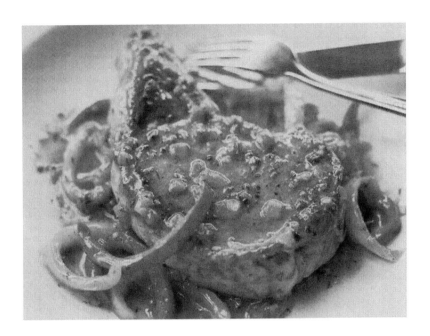

- Spread mustard on 4 pork chops and sauté both sides in oil.

- Add 250ml (8fl oz.) cider and a little brown sugar, cook a little longer then remove the chops.

- Stir in 2 tablespoons of cider vinegar, reduce and pour over the chops.

Cook for another 5 minutes.

Your Own Unique Mustard

- Create your own unique mustard by using 2 to 4 tablespoons mustard (dry or from a jar), 2 tablespoons honey and up to 1 tablespoon of vinegar (flavored or not) to create a taste and texture of your choice. Experiment by adding powdered ginger, garlic and salt. Heat to blend. Add a spoonful of flour if you need to thicken the mixture.

Try This Instead

- Try cider or malt vinegar instead of ketchup with fries. Either one is great on fish or any fried or broiled meat.

- Use up little packages or last bits of ketchup, mustard, soya sauce and other bottled sauces by mixing them with some vinegar, and adding onion, garlic and herbs of your choice to make a marinade.

- Cider vinegar and distilled white vinegar are strong tasting. Experiment with different kinds of vinegars in the stores to find your favorite. Rice wine vinegar, rice vinegar and many other flavored types of vinegar are "softer" and may be used in most recipes. Refrigerate.

Sardines In Vinegar

- Gently fry floured sardines in olive oil, then dry and lay in a dish.

- Simmer a marinade of 3 parts good red wine vinegar to 1 part water, plus bay leaves, coriander seeds, garlic and teaspoon of sugar.

When cool, pour over the fish and pop in the fridge.

Vinegar Pie

- Line a 9-inch tin with pastry and bake covered

- Add 450g (1Ib) of sugar and 55g (20z) of flour to 450ml (16fl oz.) of boiling water and cook for 5 minutes

- Away from heat, whisk in 2 beaten eggs.

- Back on the heat; beat in 6 tablespoons cider vinegar and a dash of Limón cello. Cool and refrigerate till set.

Get Rid Of Kitchen Odors

Cooking Smells And Smoke

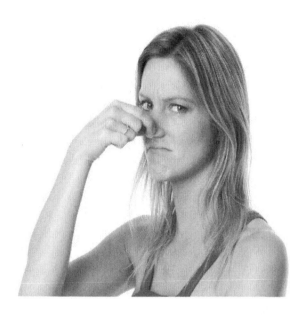

A habitually challenging task is trying to clean the air of stale smoke and food scents: conventional chemical room fresheners simply mask the smell and are often overwhelming in them. Worse still, they basically yell out loud that your home smells and you have tried to hide the fact! Use simple solutions to deal with them.

- For fish odor: place a few bowls of white vinegar around the house, odors will disappear in a day.

- Preparing fish and strong smelling produce like garlic and onions can make both hands and cooking surfaces smelly. White vinegar will remove the smells from surfaces, nevertheless, before you start preparing any fish or cut vegetables, try wiping your hands with vinegar first. It'll make it less difficult to remove the smell afterwards.

- Remove kitchen scents that come from pots or when cooking specific vegetables by bringing to a boil a modest amount of water with 1 / 4 cup vinegar so the steam circulates within the chamber. Add a few shakes of cinnamon or pot-pourri to the water for additional perfume.

Vinegar As Salad Dressings

Experiment with different types of vinegars in the shops to locate your favorite. Distilled white vinegar and cider vinegar are strong tasting. Rice wine vinegar, rice vinegar and several other flavored vinegars are softer and can be used in any recipe in which you prefer.

The basic vinaigrette salad dressing:

- 1 tablespoon of vinegar to 4 tablespoons oil, or 1/2 cup vinegar to 2 cups of oil

- Adding 1/3 to 1/4 teaspoon salt into a vinegar cruet will give a bit of seasoning and keep the vinegar clear.

- Place some balsamic vinegar that has a much more intense flavor and will be higher-priced, in a clear glass spray bottle. Now it's simpler to dispense small amounts.

- Create your own flavorful citrus vinaigrette by first combining 1) part balsamic vinegar with 2 parts olive oil. To that add 1 teaspoon sugar, 1 teaspoon mustard, 1 crushed garlic clove and orange juice equal to the quantity of the vinegar used. Lemon juice may be utilized in place of orange juice.

- Make a creamy vinaigrette by adding some plain or whipped cream into a combination of 1) part vinegar to 3 parts oil.

- Create delicious and captivating vinaigrette with zing by combing in a blender or food processor: 1/4 cup raspberry vinegar, 1/2 cup olive oil, 1/4 cup water, a garlic clove and 1-8 oz. jar of pickled beets, drained.

Kitchen Accident Tips

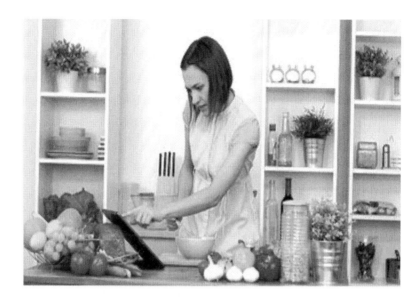

- Save money by replacing 1 teaspoon vinegar for every single teaspoon of lemon called for in any recipe. Obviously in case you really want the flavor of the lemon, this will definitely not work well.

- Perk up any can of soup or sauce with a teaspoon of red or white wine vinegar.

- Remove smells of mayo or peanut-butter in jars you have washed and desire to save by rinsing with vinegar.

- Relieve thirst by drinking a spoonful or two of apple cider vinegar in a glass of "really" cold water.

- Add a tablespoon to 1/4 cup white vinegar to soup stock you're preparing, in order to pull every bit of calcium in the bones as they cook down.

- If you added too much salt to a recipe by mistake: simple add a spoonful of vinegar and sugar to try correcting the taste.

- Avoid the oily taste in food cooked in a deep fryer with the addition of a dash of vinegar.

- You have burned yourself in the kitchen? Pour a touch of white vinegar on a small fabric and lay it around the bottom.

Flavored Vinegars

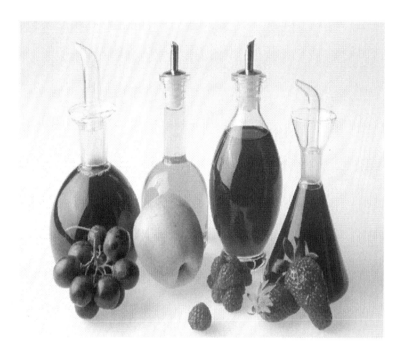

Lately there's been a burst of flavored vinegars available in the market. Particularly with balsamic vinegar of which there are currently varieties featuring herbs and flowers.

Although considered as wine vinegar, it is in fact generated from grape pressings that haven't been permitted to ferment into wine. It's rich, smooth depth of taste is imparted to the food when used in cooking.

How To Make Flavored Vinegar

Creating your own flavored vinegar is easy. White vinegar is frequently used as a base, because its clarity and high acid content will complement the variety of added ingredients. Rice vinegar and apple cider vinegars are often used as well. You may use leaves of herbs or sprigs, hot peppers, raw garlic to create your own flavors.

If you choose to use fruits like raspberries, it is essential that you first cook down the fruit adding a tbsp. of honey or sugar to the mixture before pouring it into a wide mouth jar of your choice and then cover it with vinegar.

Cool, cap and label, and give it a week or two before tasting. Flavored vinegars should last no less than 2 years when stored in a cool dry area. Berry fruits can alter color but they do not spoil as the vinegar is a safe preservative.

- Make your very own hot vinegars by carefully warming 1qt of vinegar to which you've added dry spices such as cinnamon sticks, peppercorns or whole cloves. Wait until the vinegar is cooled then strain, bottle and label.

- Put your peeled cloves of garlic from a whole garlic bulb in a quart glass jar. Fill it with white vinegar or white wine vinegar and let this sit covered tightly for at least 2 weeks. If you only have a metal jar lid, put a small plastic sandwich bag underneath the lid so the vinegar will not come in contact with it. It will have a powerful garlic taste. One teaspoon garlic powder will replace for 1 garlic clove.

- Lavender vinegar is created with unseasoned rice vinegar using a few sprigs of lavender, left to stand, and covered, for a couple of weeks. This type of vinegar is not for contributing to food but to utilize as a warm fragrant, deodorizer or cleaning product.

- Sterilize new containers that you're using for flavored vinegars to stop the vinegars from clouding.

- Make your own portion of wine vinegar by adding a tablespoon of white or red wine to two tablespoons of white vinegar. If you desire to make a larger amount use 1/4 to 1/2 cup of red or white wine to 1 cup of white vinegar or cider vinegar.

- Use rose petals or any sweet smelling flower to give a wonderful aroma to some white vinegar.

How To Use Flavored Vinegars

- Make a fast vegetable or cracker dip by combining 4 tablespoons mayo with 1 teaspoon of your flavored vinegar of choice.

- Save the juice from fish cooked in vinegar and add a little to some basic vinaigrette. Use it on the salad you serve with the fish for a complementary taste.

- Add a touch of any herb flavored vinegar when making tuna salad.

- Give a new flavor to your favorite potato salad recipe calling for white vinegar by using an herb flavored or seasoned rice one in its place.

- Make marinated mushrooms that have been rinsed and stems trimmed by first bringing them to a boil and simmering in a sauce pan for 10 minutes: 3/4 cup vegetable or olive oil, 1/2 cup of an herb flavored vinegar, 1 teaspoon salt, 1 teaspoon sugar, 1 bay leaf and a few peppercorns. Put in one pound or so of mushrooms and simmer for 3 minutes uncovered. Put mushrooms and fluid into a pan. Cover and cool for several hours or overnight. Remove bay leaf and peppercorns and drain mushrooms.

Flavored Vinegar Recipes

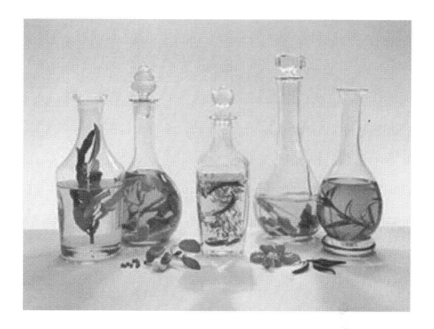

Rosemary Vinegar

Makes 2 cups

One pound of fresh rosemary sprigs. Two cups white wine or cider vinegar.

This recipe can be used with many different herbs - try using:

- thyme
- tarragon
- bay
- marjoram

The more delicate herbs for example basil, dill, coriander and mint will need their leaves bruising a little. Avoid using dried herbs or spices since these could make the vinegar cloudy for maximum flavor.

- Remove the woody stems from the rosemary and place half in a glass bowl. Pour over the vinegar, stir and then cover lightly, leave in a cool area for 7 days stirring occasionally.

- Strain, discarding the rosemary. Repeat with all the remaining rosemary and pour the strained vinegar over. Cover lightly and stir occasionally afterward leave for a further 7 days. Add 2-3 rinsed sprigs of fresh rosemary and screw down tightly.

Keep in a dark place.

Spiced Vinegar

Makes 4 pints/3 cups

6 tsps. peppercorns
3 tsps. mustard seeds
2 tsps. allspice
1 blade mace
1 large cinnamon stick, bruised
4 fresh bay leaves
1 small piece of root ginger. Chopped
1 tbsp. salt
3 cups malt vinegar

This is ideal if you desire to make your own chutneys and pickles, You can alter the spices used according to your preferred taste, White distilled vinegar is frequently used since it provides a sharper tang, however white wine, red or malt vinegar is great to use too.

Tie all of the spices into a piece of muslin cloth and place in a nonreactive saucepan. Add 1 cup of the Vinegar and bring to the boil. Boil for 3 minutes then add the remaining Vinegar and boil for a further 3 minutes. Remove from the heat and leave covered for at least 24 hours. Strain into sterilized bottles and screw down.

Raspberry Vinegar

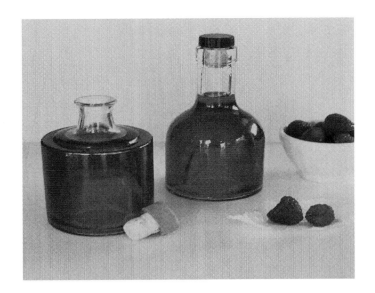

Perfect for mixed greens or fruit salads

Bruise 1 cup fresh raspberries and put them in a sanitized vessel.

- Heat wine vinegar or white to below the boiling point.
- Pour the vinegar in the vessel and cover tightly.

Leave for two to three weeks.

Lemon Thyme Vinegar

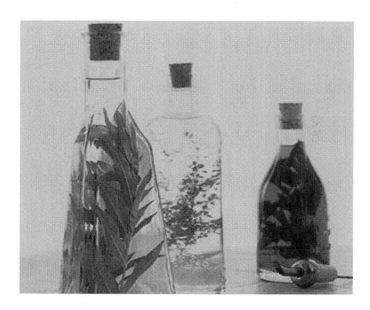

- Peel one lemon in a thin spiral (removing the colored part only) and put in a sanitized jar with four to five springs of lemon thyme or thyme.

- Heat the white vinegar below boiling point.

- Pour vinegar in a jar and cover tightly.

Leave for three to four weeks.

Remove peel and thyme then Strain vinegar. Put the vinegar in a clean jar, adding peel and fresh thyme sprigs for garnish. Seal tightly.

Orange Mint Vinegar

Use in dressing for tossed green salads with orange and grapefruit sections or in marinades for chicken or lamb chops.

- Peel one medium orange in a very thin spiral (removing the colored part only) and put in a sanitized jar.

- Gentle bruise 1/2 cup freshly mints leaves and add to jar.

- Heat white vinegar or apple cider to below boiling point.

- Pour the vinegar into a jar and cover tightly.

Leave for three to four weeks. Remove mint and peel then strain vinegar. Put the vinegar in a clean jar, adding peel and fresh mint for garnish. Cover tightly.

Basil Garlic Vinegar

Use in dressings for rice, pasta, antipasto salads or in flavored mayonnaise.

- Put 1/2 teacup crudely cut fresh basil leaves and two cloves of garlic, peeled and split, in a sanitized jar.

- Heat white vinegar or wine vinegar boiling point.

- Fill the jar with vinegar and cover tightly.

Leave for three to four weeks. Uncap, strain vinegar and discard garlic and basil. Put the vinegar into a sterilized jar; add a little fresh basil to garnish. Cover tightly.

CHAPTER 2

VINEGAR IN YOUR KITCHEN

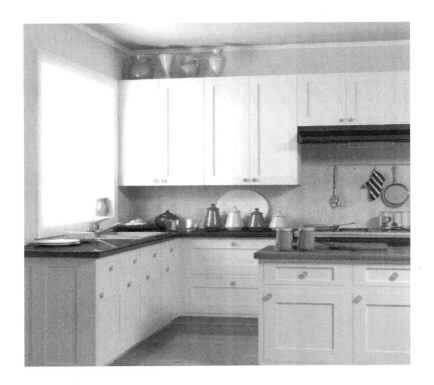

Vinegar works wonders within the kitchen and can be utilized for everything from cleaning the pot to cleaning up your waste-disposal unit. As new supplies for cookware and kitchen utensils come on to the marketplace, it's usually best to test the vinegar first on a tiny area only to be certain the material from which it's made will react as needed to the vinegar.

Then you can start cleaning away. Scents abound in kitchen areas and sometimes these can become overpowering. A straightforward remedy is to keep a small bowl half-filled with vinegar to deodorize the place.

Sink Tips

A waste disposal unit is a beneficial gadget to have in the kitchen, but, the unit may become incredibly smelly.

An easy tip would be to pour equal amounts of vinegar and bicarbonate of soda to the empty disposal unit, leave for ten minutes then flush through with clean water.

You can try this instead; freeze vinegar into ice cubes within an ice cube tray and, from time to time, drop several cubes to the disposal unit. Then change the unit on with just a small amount of cold running water and the odors will vanish.

Make certain you flush the unit through finally with clean water, remembering that vinegar can corrode some metals. Your drain itself collects all types of food garbage, oil and general gunk from washing dishes.

To remove grime build-up, pour full-strength vinegar on to the area and leave for a couple minutes. A quick scrub will shift the dirt but do not forget the all-important final rinse with clean warm water. To clean the sink's surface, a wipe down with a cloth dipped in vinegar will leave it sparkling like new once more.

Use Vinegar To Clean Glassware

You can make your cloudy glasses clear once again by soaking them for 15 - 20 minutes in a solution of white vinegar and equal parts hot water and scrub with a soft bottle brush.

Coffee and tea stained mugs and cups can be easily be restored by scrubbing with equal parts vinegar and salt followed by a rinse in warm water.

Cutting Boards

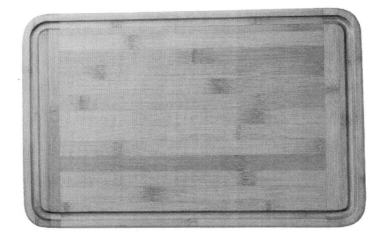

The tendency to use plastic chopping boards in place of wood is primarily because of the risk of infection which will originate from germs lurking in the grooves and cuts within the wood.

Cleaning them is not a hard job if you use vinegar, in the event you go for wooden boards. Wash the board with warm water then wipe it with full strength vinegar, after you have prepared your meal. This will kill any bacteria that may be there.

Can Openers

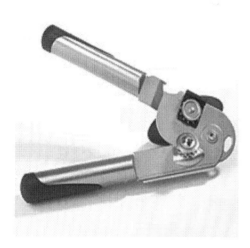

Are you horrified from the quantity of muck that is lurking there? Every time you open a can some of that muck will end up deposited on the surface of the food inside the can. Clean and disinfect your can opener by scrubbing the mechanism with a re-cycled toothbrush and immersing it in undiluted white Vinegar.

Grease Stains

Sprinkle vinegar on fish and chips to cut through the grease making the food easier to digest. Damp a cloth in equal parts of white wine vinegar and water to tackle grease marks. Not only can it get rid of the grease, the vinegar will also remove any lingering greasy odors.

Grill Pans

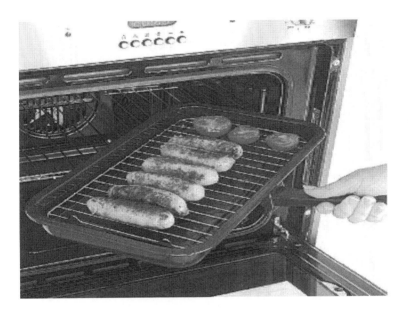

It's the grease which has dripped from food into the grill pan that smells when you heat the grill up. Too much gathered grease in a grill pan can also catch fire. Lining the pan with cooking foil is one way of keeping a watch on things, but even then you still need to clear out the pan to remove odors, splatters, spill and bacteria.

Disinfect Dishcloths

Cleaning a surface is useless in the event the dishcloth, sponge or brush is dirty; Soak them after each use in white vinegar and hot water for some minutes, then rinse and leave to dry.

Still, you can soak loofahs and natural bath sponges in-vinegar to clean them of soap residue, Rinse them off with clean water then restore them with a soak in a saltwater solution (which removes any 'slime') before giving them a another rinse in cold water.

Use Vinegar To Clean And Deodorize A Drain

Pour in one cup of hot vinegar then one cup of baking soda to deodorize any drain. Let it sit for at least 5 minutes, then run hot water down the drain.

Add 1/2 cup of hot vinegar and then 1/2 cup of baking soda to clean and deodorize any garbage disposal. Another great way to deodorize and clean garbage disposal is to use vinegar ice cubes.

Pour a few cubes of vinegar down the disposal and at the same time flushing with some cold water. As the vinegar freezes it will deodorize the freezer as well. To make vinegar ice cubes freeze vinegar in a molded ice cube tray.

Clean And Deodorize Food Containers

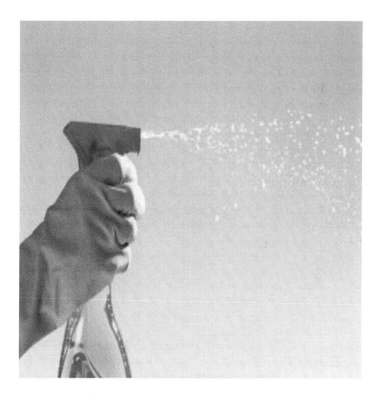

Wash food containers in a solution of equal parts white vinegar as well as water, and then rinse clean. Store with the lid off. If odors persist, place a slice of bread soaked in white vinegar within the food container (lid on) overnight: the smell should have gone by the following day.

Berry Stains

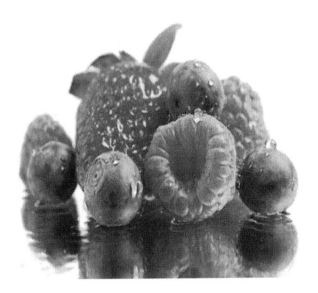

Preparing soft fruits can leave your hands and surfaces - stained. Remove stains by washing surfaces, bowls and hands with white vinegar and rinsing well with water afterwards.

Appliance

- Wash appliance exteriors with a mixture of 1/2 cup baking soda, 1/2 cup vinegar, 1 cup ammonia and a gallon of hot water.

Microwave And Fridge

- Combine and mix 1/2 cup of water and 1/2 cup vinegar in a microwave dish or glass to clean the microwave oven. Mixing cup and bringing it to a boil so the inside streams up. Odors will vanish.

- Mix a tbsp. of vinegar along with a drop or two of liquid dish soap using a cup of water and bring it to a boil in the microwave. Leave it for approximately fifteen minutes before wiping clean.

- Use half and half solution of water and vinegar to clean the shelves and walls of fridge.

Kettle De-Scalar

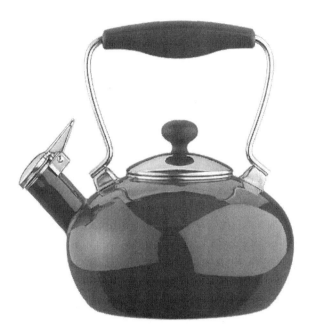

Lime and mineral deposits which have built up in coffee makers and in kettles - can be removed by boiling enough white vinegar to fill the pot to 3 / 4 full for five minutes.

Leave the Vinegar in the pot or coffee maker overnight then rinse out with cool water the next morning, rinse the kettle and fill with clean water again. Then bring to the boil. Rinse the kettle once more and your kettle will now be nice and clean again.

Coffee-Maker

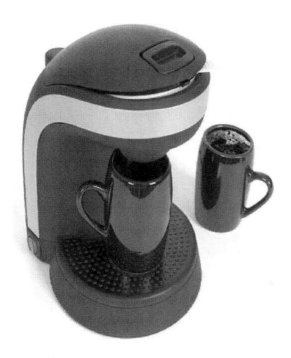

Your coffee-maker is destined to develop mineral deposits. Coffee grinds will build up through several brews, plus a brownish, muddy sludge will accumulate on the bottom and sides.

Clean by filling the pot with full strength vinegar and proceed with a regular brewing cycle. When finished, do the same again, this time using clean water. If you use a coffee pot that you simply boil on the cooker, you may use the same strategy but use equal parts vinegar and water and ensure to flush it out twice with clean water to remove any taste of vinegar.

Vinegar On Pots And Pans

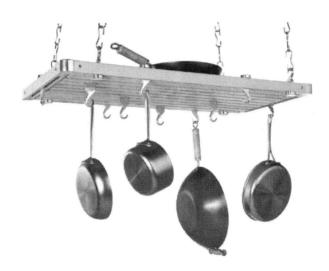

- For brass, mix and combine into a small paste of equal portions of flour and salt with sufficient vinegar and spread on to obtain the desired consistency.

- You can also perform the same job on copper pots by spraying with a mixture of hot vinegar plus a tablespoon or 2 of salt to the pot, then rinse and dry.

- For cooking pots, tarnished brass, copper, and pewter use a paste with identical amounts of table salt and vinegar for cleaning.

- Boil into a pot a mixture of one cup of water and one cup white vinegar to get rid of dark spots on aluminum pot.

Vinegar On Containers

- Add equal parts of baking soda (or salt) and vinegar using a sponge or brush, scrubbing them lightly to get rid of stains from coffee and tea cups.

- Clean a thermos by filling it with 1/4 cup white vinegar and then hot tap water. Utilize a bottle brush or fabric to whisk the insides before rinsing it clean.

- Get rid of odors from any lunch box by enclosing within it a vinegar-soaked slice of fresh bread and leaving it overnight.

- Clean a bread box and dispose of this rancid scent by wiping it out using a cloth dampened with vinegar.

CHAPTER 3

VINEGAR IN YOUR BATHROOM

Toilet Bowls Tips

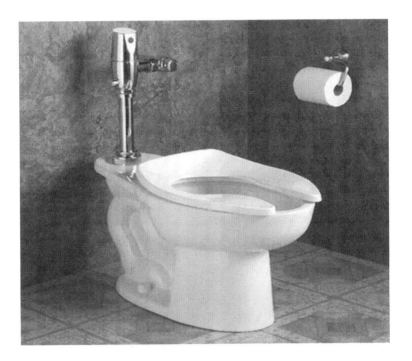

An effective and efficient method to help keep your toilet bowl disinfected without using dangerous substances will be to pour about 2 1/2 cups white vinegar slowly over the sides of the bowl before you go to bed at nights, treatment once a week should help keep away those marks that appear only above the water line in the bowl.

Add one cup borax and one cup vinegar in the bowl of the toilet. Leave it for a few minutes before using the toilet brush to wash the bowl and upward under the rim.

Freshen air in the bathroom by simple spraying into the air a solution of 1 teaspoon baking soda and 1 teaspoon vinegar and 1 cup water. Shake the squirt bottle well after the mixture stops foaming.

Shiny Showers Tips

After you take a shower, wipe down the shower glass using a solution of identical parts water and white vinegar, finally, remove all traces of vinegar and water with a sponge, and leave the shower door open to air dry.

Spray shower doors with full strength of white vinegar to prevent this from happening again after you have squeegeed the glass, which is helpful to do after each shower. It helps release the hard water deposits so that they cannot remain on the glass.

Shower Curtains Tips

Alter a shower; open the shower curtain across the railing to allow it to dry off. If the curtain has been stained by mildew, wash it in hot water with identical parts laundry detergent and bicarbonate of soda, and then rinse with 1/2 cup of white vinegar added to the rinse water.

Tiles Tips

Bring gloomy tiles back to life by washing then with a solution of 1/2 cup white vinegar in 4 cups warm water.

Use Vinegar To Unclog Plugholes

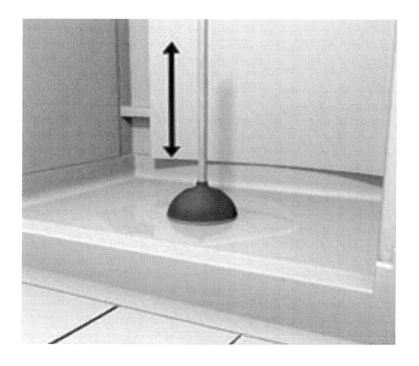

If not flushed through, soap and shower gel residues can build up inside the plug hole - more so in case that there are hairs in there too. Use a funnel and pour 4-5 tablespoons bicarbonate of soda into the plughole. Then pour in 1/2 cup white vinegar and wait until it foam and fizz.

Flush through with really hot water, when the fizzing stops. Wait five minutes then flush through with cold water. As well as clearing the blockage, you have also killed and flushed away any odor creating bacteria which were hiding there.

Grout Tips

Tile grout loses its whiteness and turns grey with age and grime over time, its rough surface and porous nature also makes it an ideal home for bacteria to grow. Use an old toothbrush dipped in white vinegar will whiten the grout, and kill germs.

Sinks and Tubs Tips

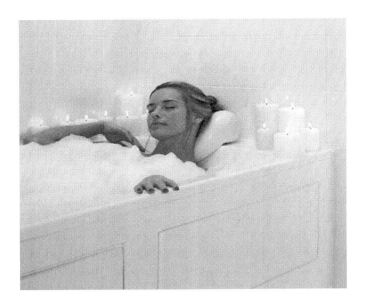

- Remove tide marks in your basin or tub by filling it with hot-water to a level just over the mark and including a generous amount of white vinegar. Leave it to soak for several hours.

Drain away the water and the marks ought to be considerably easier to clean away.

- Clean grout by allowing full strength vinegar sit on it for some minutes and scrubbing it with an old toothbrush. Bleach is, in addition, powerful however there are times you may not wish to use it.

- Kill germs all around the bathroom with a spray of full strength vinegar. Wipe clean with a moist cloth.

- Shine up colored porcelain sinks by scouring them with undiluted white vinegar.

Shower Heads And Taps Tips

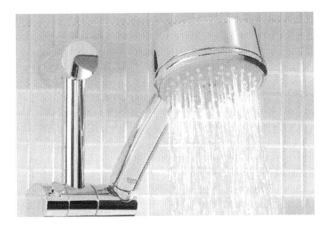

- Lime scale deposits can easily clog up the holes in shower heads: this means that water can puts pressure in your hot water system and it back up in your pipes. Handheld shower heads can be immersed easily in hot water and deep bowl of white vinegar, leave on. The vinegar will change and dissolve the mineral deposits.

- Fixed shower heads, tub and basin faucets. Fill a plastic bag with white vinegar and fasten it with cord, tape and rubber bands on the shower head. This works for faucets too, but you could also attempt fixing a plastic cup on the end. Allow the tap to sit in the vinegar for one hour, and then rinse off with a little cold water. The build-up from the hard water will be removed.

- Put a clogged, detachable showerhead in a pot full of identical portions of vinegar and water for 5 to 20 minutes. Remember to get rid of the rubber washer first.

CHAPTER 4

ALL-PURPOSE SOLUTIONS IN THE HOUSE

Remove Wax And Polish Build-up Tips

Remove polish or wax builds up on surfaces easily with a combination of identical proportions of water and white vinegar. Dip a material into the mix and wring it out well, clean off the polish. Wipe dry with a soft clean fabric.

Walls And Woodwork Tips

- Use undiluted vinegar on a fabric by wiping down walls to get rid of dust, stale smells and mildew.

- Use a combination of one cup vinegar, one cup baking soda, 1/2 cup ammonia and one gallon warm water to clean walls and woodwork. Wipe on with a sponge. Wood finishes are different and this may not be suitable for specific woods, such as on fine furniture. If uncertain, I suggest testing a small area first.

- Get rid of cloudiness on varnished wood with a solution of one quart warm water and one tbsp. white vinegar. Rub on with soft, lint less fabric, then wipe with a clean, dry fabric.

Scratches On Wooden Surfaces Tips

Small scrapes on wooden surfaces can be disguised using a small white or apple cider vinegar mixed in a jar with some iodine. Correct the color to complement the wood - more vinegar for light woods, more iodine for dark woods - and paint the scrape mark attentively with a small paint brush.

Water Rings Tips

Get rid of white ring marks on wooden table with a combination of equal portions of olive oil and vinegar by applying it with a soft material. Do not rub in circles, but move the material along the grain of the wood. Use a second clean material to polish up to a glow.

Furniture Tips

- Create an effective and frugal furniture polish with identical parts white vinegar and vegetable oil, constantly rubbing with the grain of the wood. This same remedy will often remove white water rings from wood.

- Ugly white water marks on leather furniture can be removed by dabbing them with a sponge dipped in undiluted white vinegar. Leather which has lost its radiance may be revitalized with a mixture of equal parts of white vinegar and boiled linseed oil.

- Put the solution into a spray bottle and spray on the leather. Distribute it over the top lightly with a soft material and give it two minutes to nourish the leather, and then buff using a clean material.

Leather topped tables are best cleaned by wiping with a soft material dipped in a solution of two parts water and 1 part white vinegar and dried off with a soft clean material.

Windows Tips

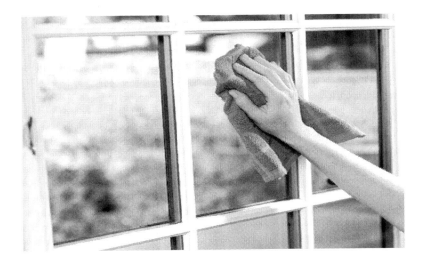

This is a tested and trusted system to get windows and mirrors very clean. Combine equal parts of water and white vinegar in a spray bottle. Spray on the glass and clean off the soil with newspaper. Finish with a mild shine with some brown paper.

Paint on Windows Tips

Dried-on paint on windows sometimes can be difficult to get rid of without scratching the glass. The easy alternative is to 'paint' on undiluted hot white vinegar onto the mark and give it time to soften up before scraping off using a razor edged tool.

Piano Keys Tips

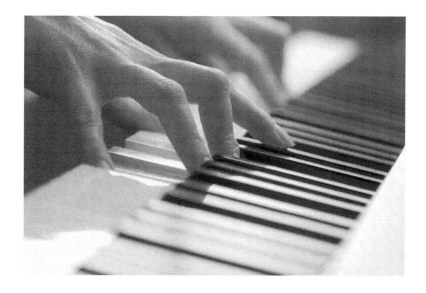

Clean piano keys with a soft material barely dampened with a mild solution of 1/2 cup vinegar to 2 cups warm water. Wring the cloth practically dry before wiping the keys clean.

Doorknobs Tips

Get rid of bacteria by spraying full strength vinegar on doorknobs and then wipe them dry. This can be mainly helpful during the flu season.

Carpet Stains Tips

- Place about 1 / 4 cup vinegar in a steam cleaner to lessen soap bubbles, and use exactly the same amount in water to eliminate detergent residue and make rugs stay clean and fresh longer.

- Clean indoor / outdoor carpeting outside using a solution of 1 cup vinegar to a bucket of hot water. Scrub it with a brush and then hose it off.

- Certain carpet stains are possible to remove by using a paste made from 4 tablespoons bicarbonate of soda and 2 tablespoons white vinegar. First test on a small area of the carpet for color fastness, and when it's secure, gently work the paste to the stained region: don't rub outwards because this can disperse the stain, rather work in the border of the stain to the center. Allow the paste to dry.

- Eliminate a non-oily spot when you detect it using a solution of a teaspoon each of vinegar plus a light liquid detergent into a gallon of hot-water. Apply and rub in with a soft brush. Rinse with clean water and blot dry. Repeat if necessary.

Vinyl and Leno Floors Tips

- Bring the glow back to your vinyl flooring without making it slippery by washing it using a solution of l/2 cup of white vinegar to every 4 liter pail of plain water. Many stains can be safely taken off linoleum floor covering by adding a splash of white vinegar, sprinkling bicarbonate of soda on the top and rubbing lightly. Rinse clean with water subsequently.

- Clean any flooring that can be cleaned using a wet solution with a mixture of two gallons water, 1 /2 capful liquid soap and one cup vinegar. Wipe the floor dry with a soft material in the event you want to get the loosened dirt.

- Add a cup of vinegar to the rinse water after scrubbing the floor using a floor stripper. This can neutralize chemicals and make the finish stick better.

Fireplace

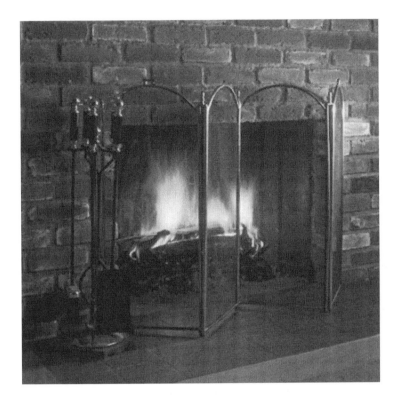

Clean your fireplace glass doors with a portion of one part vinegar to two parts water. Wipe on or spray, and then wipe clean with a dry fabric. Or scrub fireplace bricks with undiluted vinegar to get rid of grime and soot. Use a brush to scrub and a towel to blot up the dirt and wetness.

Pet Stain

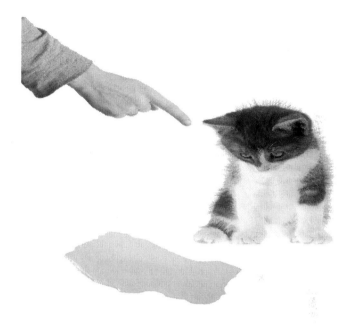

Pets will always be pets regardless. I have had several pets over the years and I loved them like my children no matter what they did, it's that cute look on their face that makes you just want to cuddle them even after their little accident. To get rid of your pet stains; start by blotting up the area and then add half and half water and vinegar solution to the area. When the area is almost dry; scatter baking soda over the area and allow drying.

CHAPTER 5

LAUNDRY - STAIN AND ODOR REMOVAL

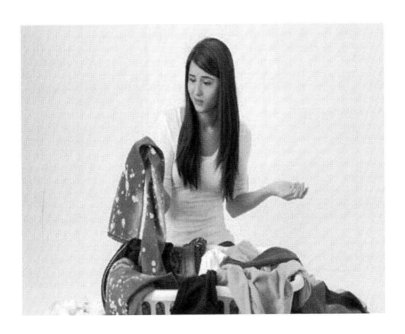

The amount of acetic acid in distilled or white vinegar is strong enough to dissolve the alkalis in detergents and soaps, but not strong enough to harm materials. Additionally, it has bactericidal properties.

White vinegar is helpful for retaining colors quickly in garments and linens. It's also a wonderful way to put the 'bounce' back into fibers as it behaves like a fabric conditioner. The acidic nature of the vinegar cuts through grease as well as the alkalis that form the bottom of several soaps and detergents.

Ink Spots Tips

Treat the ink stain first by blotting with undiluted white vinegar, and then gently rub in a paste of 2 parts white vinegar and 3 parts corn flour. Allow the paste to dry fully on the ink stain, blot and then launder as usual.

Pre-Wash Stain Removal Tips

White vinegar is such a useful pre wash stain remover. As you check over garments before putting them in the washer, treat any heavy grime or underarm perspiration stains with a quick spray of vinegar of half-and-half solution of white vinegar and water.

- Soap residue makes black garments look dull. Add vinegar to your final rinse to remove soap residue.

- Use your bleach or fabric softener dispenser to hold vinegar to the wash cycle and when you wish to flush these dispensers clean.

Collars And Cuffs Tips

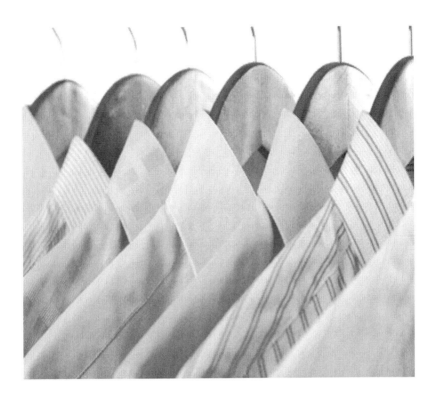

Collars and cuffs are especially exposed to stain, particularly oily ones from perfumes and makeup. Create a paste of 2 parts white vinegar and 3 parts bicarbonate of soda and utilize a soft nail brush - or a waste and recycled toothbrush - to lightly brush the paste in to the cuffs and collars. Allow the paste set on the cloth for 30 minutes and then launder as usual.

Deodorant Stains Tips

Deodorants and Antiperspirants can leave nasty white marks on clothes. These can be removed by lightly rubbing white vinegar on them and then laundering as usual.

Bloodstains Tips

Bloodstains are rather simple to remove before they have dried and set into cloth but are virtually impossible to remove after 24 hours. Pour undiluted white vinegar directly on the area, if you're able to get to the bloodstain fast and allow it to soak in for 5 - 10 minutes before blotting with a clean material. Repeat if needed and then launder as usual.

Unset Old Stains Tips

Older unset stains can be effectively removed by treating the affected area with a solution of 3 tablespoons white vinegar, 2 tablespoons liquid detergent and 4 1/2 cups warm water. Repeatedly sponge and blot the area then launder.

Bring Your Vintage Lace Back To Its Former Glory

Old and classic lace is often quite fine, so start any cleaning procedure by soaking it first in cold water and allowing it dry naturally. Use a really light solution of water and white vinegar, 24 parts water and one part white vinegar for an overnight soak, if it's still in the yellow side when dry.

Rinse well and allow the lace to dry naturally (in the sunlight) if possible, because this can also assist in the 'bleaching' procedure.

Wine Stains Tips

Wine stains can be taken out from cotton and cotton polyester fabrics - but only in the event you get to the stain in a period of 24 hours.

Use undiluted white vinegar: sponge it softly on to the area and blot using a clean material. Repeat until as much of the wine stain has been removed and then wash according to the care label directions for the garment.

Use This Instead Of Bleach

Your dull socks can be brighter! Get back the color in your dull white socks by adding 7 1/4 cups cold water and about 2/3 cups white vinegar into a sizable container and bring it to the boil. Place the socks into a pail and pour the boiling vinegar solution over them, allow it to soak overnight and the following day, launder them as usual.

Restore Whites Tips

- Use vinegar on mildewed garments that can't take bleach.

- Scrub a paste of vinegar and baking soda on ring-around the-collar before tops go into the washer.

- Keep bright colors from bleeding during washing by soaking items in a solution of 1 cup vinegar and 1 gallon water before washing.

- Bring out brilliant colors by adding 1/2 cup vinegar to the rinse cycle.

Odor Removal

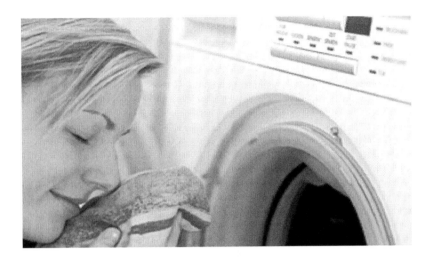

Get Rid Of Smells From Clothes Tips

- Remove perspiration odor and spots on garments, as well as those left by deodorants, by spraying full strength vinegar on collar and underarm areas before throwing them into the washer.

- Add 1 to 2 cups vinegar to the final rinse water for cotton or wool blankets to fluff them, also.

- Use vinegar in the rinse water for bed linens and table linens to keep them from yellowing in storage.

- When doing hand laundry add a small amount of vinegar to the last rinse to cut excess suds. Follow this with another plain rinse.

Keep Your Machine Clean

You won't get clean clothing from a dirty washing machine. Pour in about 1 cup white vinegar and run the washing machine on a complete cycle but without clothing or detergents once in a while. This can remove mineral deposits, clean out remaining soap scum and deodorize your washer.

Kill Bacteria In Washers

Due to the acetic acid content, white vinegar has bactericidal properties. Putting about 1/2 cup white vinegar to your washers rinse cycle will kill off any bacteria existing in the wash load, particularly if it has diapers. White vinegar will normally break down uric acid from baby and kids clothes.

Suede Stains Tips

Grease marks on shoes and purses as well as suede garments can be easily eliminated if you dip a clean toothbrush into white vinegar and lightly brush the mark, don't scrub! Or you'll damage the nap, allow the mark to air dry then brush with a suede brush and repeat if needed. Make your suede items look good as new by gentle wiping around using a sponge dipped in white vinegar.

Say Good Bye To Fabric Softeners

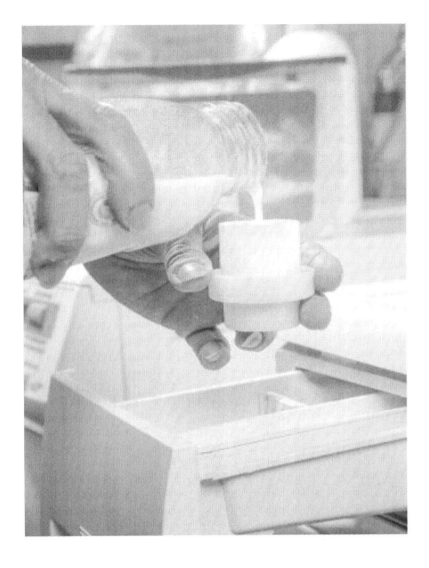

If you don't want your laundry smelling of artificial perfumes, there isn't any need for expensive fabric softening liquids. Instead, try adding 1/2 cup white vinegar for the final rinse for soft and fresh smelling clothes.

Salt Marks Tips

A quick fix for winter

Boots and shoes are easily spoiled in the winter. As soon as you can wipe off fresh salt stains on boots and shoes with a sponge dipped in undiluted white vinegar and allow drying.

Blanket Reviver

Wool, cotton blankets and bedding can be revived and made fluffy and soft as well as free of soap deposits and odors by adding about 1 cup white vinegar for the last rinse cycle.

Keep Woollens in Shape

Make a solution of 1 part white vinegar to 2 parts warm water and soak for 20 to 25 minutes, gently squeeze out the excess water, but don't wring the garment as you'll just twist the yam and extend it further.

When you've squeezed most of the water out, layout the fabric flat on a large folded up towel and gently arrange the fabric back to fit, Place another towel on top and gently blot, letting the towels absorb more wetness, Place the clothing flat on a dry towel and allow it to dry naturally.

Get Rid Of Wrinkles

At times clothing get creases and wrinkles that have dried in, this can occur even if they're brand new. De-wrinkle them by hanging the garment on a clothes hanger and lightly spraying a mist of a solution of 1 part white vinegar and 3 parts water. Allow the garment to air-dry.

Color Maintenance Tips

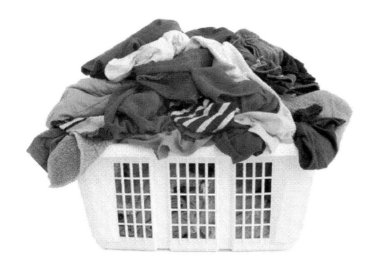

Keep Colors Fast

Old as well as new colored garments can lose a lot of their color in the wash and you will end up with bleached or streaky patches. Soak colored fabrics and garments for a couple of minutes in a bowl of diluted white Vinegar before you wash them, to repair the color.

Stop Red From Running Tips

Red colors is known for running in the wash and turning everything washed with it pink, but pre-soaking a new red item in undiluted vinegar before the first wash can restrict the amount of red dye which is shed.

It is best to wash dark and colored items separately from white items; however you will find the red items do not lose a lot of their color in the long term.

Ironing

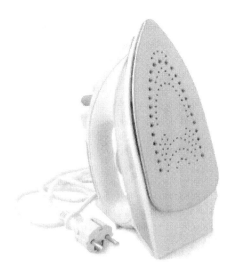

Flush Out Your Iron

- Fill the reservoir with full strength white vinegar. Set the iron in a vertical position, then switch the iron on to its steam setting, allow the vinegar steam clean the interior for ten to fifteen minutes. This will help prevent the corroding and get rid of any mineral deposits. Repeat with clean water to flush out some remaining vinegar.

- Get rid of scorch marks from an iron by rubbing it with a warmed-up solution of identical parts salt and vinegar. If that does not work, use a material dampened with full-strength vinegar.

- Wipe the underneath of your cold iron with a material soaked in full strength vinegar to eliminate any brownish residue there. Repeat as-needed.

- Remove the crease left by the old hem of the wool garment by sponging the line with full strength vinegar.

Remove Scorch Marks From Clothes

Small negligible scorch marks on clothes will frequently come out by rubbing scorch marks with a clean cloth dampened in white vinegar and then blot with a clean cloth, repeating if necessary.

CHAPTER 6

HOW TO STAY HEALTHY WITH APPLE CIDER VINEGAR

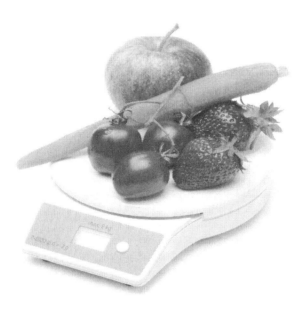

Can eating an apple a day really keep the doctor away? It can certainly help you to control your blood sugar and gain all the benefits that come with that control. In fact, researchers have found that women who eat at least one apple a day are 28 per cent less likely to develop 'Type 2 diabetes compared to those who do not eat apples.

That is probably because apples are filled with soluble fiber - the number one for blunting blood sugar level swings. A medium apple serves up an outstanding 4g of fiber, mainly pectin, which is known for its capability to reduced cholesterol.

Planning to get rid of your belly fat? (Keep in mind, stomach fat is bad for blood sugar.) Try eating three small apples each day.

A recent report from the State University of Rio de Janeiro discovered that doing so as part of a reduced-calorie diet plan not only assisted women to shed more weight but additionally helped them to reduce their blood sugar levels significantly more than women who ate another food as opposed to apples.

To get every little benefit from apples, go for whole, unpeeled good fresh fruit. The apples with the lowest GL are Brae-burns, which have more acid and not as much sugar than Golden Delicious.

Following on the scale is unsweetened apple sauce, which offers several of the exact same health and wellness benefits. However, stay away from apple juice; it's not much better than apple-flavored liquid sugar.

Like many fruits, apples include vitamins, minerals along with other antioxidant properties which may help decrease the chance of cancer by preventing DNA damage.

Boron, the mineral that is found in apples, may possibly retard bone loss in women after menopause and may help women on estrogen replacement therapy keep the estrogen in their system for much longer.

Using a suitable mix of mindful eating, plentiful exercise and apple-cider vinegar, your weight loss goals can be reachable.

Remain focused, and have patience - all it takes is a little bit of dedication. Calorie counting and exercise alone will not take off fat, but apple cider vinegar is a crucial element to make the process painless.

Not only will your blood sugar stabilize as well as your blood pressure lowered, but the appetite suppression properties of apple cider vinegar will protect you from your hunger pangs that plague most dieting hopefuls.

Regardless of your goal, if you have 10 pounds to lose or 100 apple-cider vinegar will help. Your health will enhance, and your energy will grow.

Roast Beef Recipe

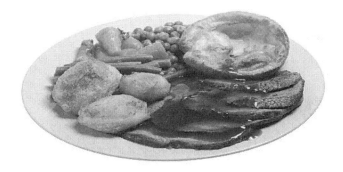

2 small onions,
sliced 2 ½ tablespoons of olive oil
1 large beef roast
1 cup organic apple cider vinegar
1 cup organic apple juice
2/ 3 cup rapadura
½ teaspoon allspice

Directions:

In an oven-proof pot with a cover, over a burner on medium-high, heat the olive oil and onions, brown the meat on all sides. Keep browning meat and turning until the onions brown as well.

Combine the vinegar, apple juice, rapadura and allspice. Remove pot from the burner, pour mixture over the beef, cover, and put in a 325 degree oven. Cook beef for about 3 hours or until tender. Turn the beef in the liquid every 10 minutes. Serve with marinated vegetables.

Delicious Chickpeas and Spinach

With Quinoa Recipe

This is one of my favorite recipe, especially when am on a cleansing diet. Spinach is very powerful and rich in chlorophyll, which helps to cleanse the blood and colon.

1 tablespoon organic apple cider vinegar
3 tablespoons expeller-pressed olive oil
1 teaspoon mustard powder
1 tablespoon raw honey
1 cup organic baby spinach
½ cup red quinoa, cooked
½ cup chickpeas, cooked
½ cup artichoke hearts, cooked
6 organic cherry tomatoes
½ of an avocado, cubed

Directions:

To prepare vinaigrette, blend vinegar, olive oil, mustard powder, and honey with a whisk. Set aside. Place baby spinach in a large serving bowl.

Mix with prepared vinaigrette. Add quinoa and mix until well incorporated. Top with chickpeas, artichoke hearts, cherry tomatoes, and avocado.

CHAPTER 7

BEAUTY AND GROOMING

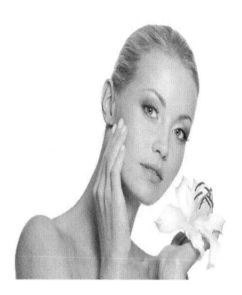

For several generations, the Japanese have recognized the advantages of vinegar as a beauty aid and, as Western consumers continue to seek skin friendly and natural treatments, vinegar sits in our cupboard as the achiever.

The styptic and toning qualities of vinegar especially apple cider vinegar have for centuries been employed as part of women's and men's beauty regimes. Vinegar is considerably more astringent than ice and will reduce redness, bruising, inflammation and swelling in about half the time.

Skin

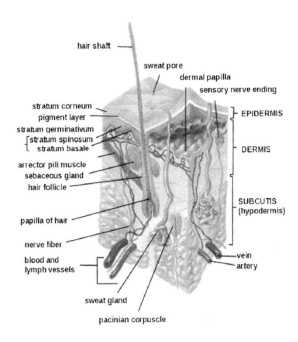

hair shaft

sweat pore

dermal papilla

sensory nerve ending

stratum corneum
pigment layer
stratum germinativum
stratum spinosum
stratum basale

EPIDERMIS

DERMIS

arrector pili muscle
sebaceous gland
hair follicle

SUBCUTIS
(hypodermis)

papilla of hair

nerve fiber

blood and
lymph vessels

vein
artery

sweat gland

pacinian corpuscle

Your Skin is profoundly influenced by the environment, diet and the pressures of day-to-day life; therefore it deserves the very best care and treatment. Vitamin C is an extremely important element for skin and, with the aid of vinegar; it is easily digested by the body.

Vinegar also helps to bring back the natural pH balance of the skin, so drink a teaspoon of apple cider vinegar in a glass of water each day.

Age Spots

Age Gracefully By Using Vinegar

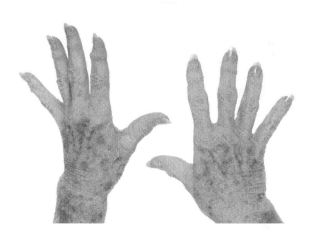

Apply full strength apple cider vinegar dabbing with a cotton pad for about ten minutes two times per day to successfully repair your hands. The spots will fade in a couple of weeks. Age spots can be caused by hormonal changes, and due to over-exposure to the sun.

Dietary Changes

- Store all seeds and nuts in the refrigerator or freezer, as they can easily become rancid. Stay away from rancid oils. Refrigerate all oils; never store them on a shelf at room temperature once opened. Grains should be stored in a cool, dry place. Stay away from all fried foods. Hot grease and cooking oils contain high amounts of skin-damaging substances.

- Stay away from junk food, tobacco caffeine, alcohol, and sweets.

- Cleanse your liver. Drink beet juice. Two or three ounces of beet juice per day will be sufficient in the beginning of your cleansing program.

As you detoxify your liver, you can increase your intake of beet juice to six ounces.

Nutrients That Helps

- Beta-carotene is an antioxidant that slows the aging process.

- Vitamin C is an antioxidant that helps in repairing tissue.

- Bioflavonoids work synergistically with vitamin C to repair tissues.

- Vitamin E is an antioxidant that reduces the aging process and helps repair tissue.

The Amazing Vinegar Peel

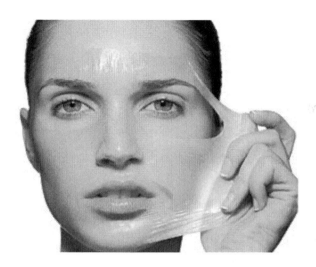

The purpose of a cosmetic peel is really to release the epidermis of the skin, eliminating a layer to expose the layer beneath. The hypothesis is the fact that the new skin encourages a fresher, younger-looking appearance but the procedure can be expensive.

This is also a gentle treatment, and if performed too harshly, faces can appear as if they can be gravely sunburned. A more affordable and simpler edition, which is often utilized for a home treatment, is the vinegar peel.

Scrub your face then apply vinegar directly on your skin; leave for five full minutes. Rinse the vinegar off and your skin will feel soft and look much fresher. Your Skin will be sensitive to sunlight, so stay out of direct sunshine for an hour after treatment.

Fix Bruises And Broken Veins

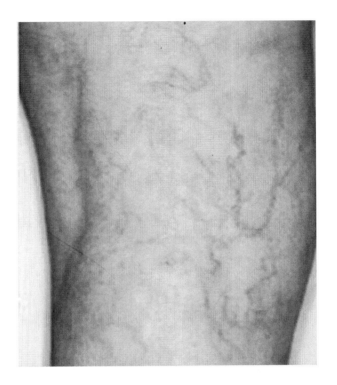

As a mild astringent, apple cider vinegar is a helpful treatment for all those miniature, but unsightly broken veins that may frequently appear on top of skin.

Dab on undiluted apple cider vinegar to reduce redness and speed up the repair once or twice a day. Bruises may also be treated in the same manner.

How To Get Rid Of Blackheads

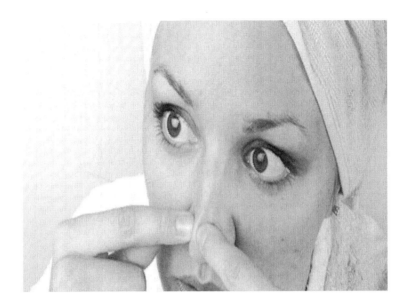

Blackheads are annoying and embarrassing, the consequence of having a greasy skin or teenage acne. The property of strawberries when combined with vinegar provides a natural deep cleanser.

Combine 1/3 cup vinegar with five chopped strawberries and leave at room-temperature for a few hours. Strain the liquid through a sieve and remove the strawberry pulp. Gentle, pat the liquid on to the area affected by blackheads before retiring to bed. Rinse off in the morning and repeat until the blackheads clear.

How To Get Rid Of Acne

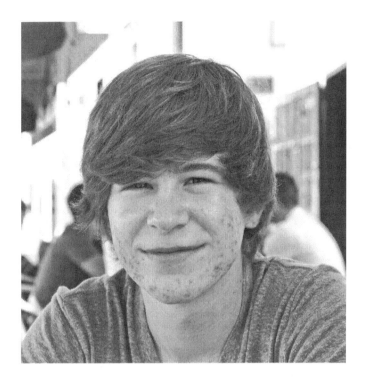

Acne is a general term often used to indicate acne vulgaris, which is a chronic inflammatory disease of the sebaceous glands and hair follicles of the skin. It is characterized by blackheads, whiteheads, and pimples. Chronic acne can result in scarring.

A contributing factor may be diet, as evidenced by studies of Eskimos and other cultures that first experienced acne after adopting the Western diet. Some acne is caused by a condition known as "skin hypoglycemia" or "skin diabetes."

This means that the skin (which is an organ) is intolerant to sugars. Acne can cause embarrassment and loss of self-esteem, and this is what every teenager's dread.

General References

Cleanse your face at least twice a day. After washing, apply benzoyl peroxide 5-percent gel at night. Extract blackheads every two or three days. Avoid using greasy creams and cosmetics, and avoid medications that contain bromides or iodides.

Dietary Changes

1. Eliminate sugars. A study has shown that skin glucose tolerance is significantly impaired in acne patients.

2. Eat a high fiber diet. Client's skin has cleared rapidly when fiber was increased in the diet. Foods high in fiber are fruits, vegetables, whole grain cereals, whole grain breads and crackers, bran, and legumes (beans, lentils, and split peas).

Nutrients That Helps

- Take Vitamin A to slow down the production of sebum. Be aware. Though, that Side effects may result from high doses of Supplemental Vitamin A. Beta-carotene, which can be found in fresh vegetables and fruits, is a smarter choice. Beta-carotene is transformed into Vitamin A as your body needs.

- For acne breakouts, take Vitamin B6. It is helpful for premenstrual acne breakouts.

- Folic Acid can be helpful also.

- Selenium with vitamin E can regularize glutathione peroxidase levels.

- Chromium increases glucose tolerance levels and improves insulin sensitivity.

- For tissue regeneration and inflammation control, Zinc plays an important role in wound healing.

- A low-fat diet can be helpful along with essential fatty acids. A good source of omega-S fatty acids is pure cold-pressed flaxseed oil and cold-water fatty fish and green vegetables.

Acne Vinegar Remedy

A good remedy that is certainly economical and easy to make is a combination of one teaspoon vinegar to ten teaspoons water. Empty it into a little, handy bottle, through the entire day, dab it on to pimples and spots.

The skin will be helped by the vinegar mixture to get back to its normal pH balance. Another home treatment is to make a paste composed of two teaspoonful apple-cider vinegar, one teaspoonful of honey and one teaspoon of flour.

Leave this on overnight and rinse off in the morning. Always test it first on a single blemish; if it is effective, the blemish should heal quicker.

How To Get Rid Of Flaking Skin And Oily Skin

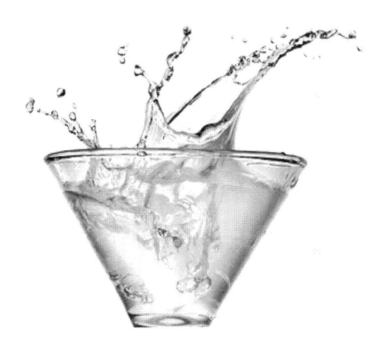

Whether the skin is greasy or dry, apple cider vinegar is rich in acids that help to dissolve fat and reduce flaking while encouraging a softer, smoother complexion.

A combination of equal parts apple cider vinegar and water placed on the face, allowed to dry, then rinsed with water will enable your skin to breath much easier and look fresher.

How To Make Your Own Night Cream

Using Apple Cider Vinegar For A Radiant Glow

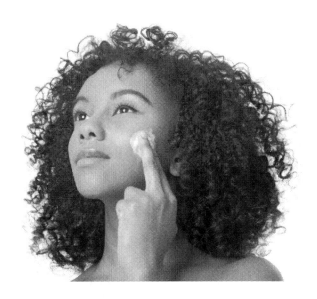

The cost of commercially skin treatments is sufficient to make you think that they work. However you can create your own natural treatments which will perform just as well.

Mix 1/2 cup olive oil with three teaspoons apple cider vinegar, diluted with enough water to create a cream. Apply small quantities to the face before bedtime and rinse off the following day with water. Your skin will feel moisturized and cleansed.

Men Can Use It Too!

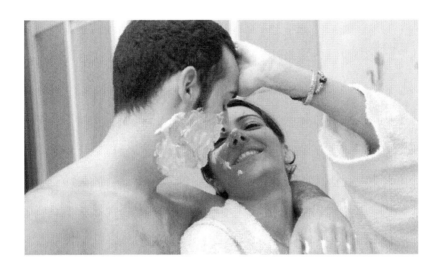

As an after-shave, small amounts of vinegar will keep the skin looking great and keep shaved skin disinfected. Use undiluted vinegar as an aftershave lotion, particularly if commercial aftershaves cause itching and rashes. Your skin will be soft, and skin problems will be helped.

- Tone facial skin using a solution of equal portions of vinegar as well as water.

- Steam clean your face using apple cider vinegar.

- Lean over a pot of boiling water (carefully at least 8-inches from the water) with a towel over your head to trap the steam. After a minute, apply apple cider vinegar

Tooth Care

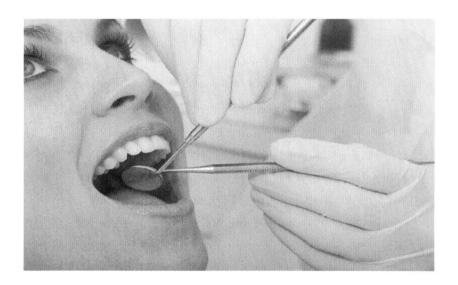

Get rid of bad breath and whiten your teeth by brushing them a couple of times per week with white vinegar. Soak dentures overnight in warm water with 1/4 cup white vinegar. This will soften tartar so that it can be easily brushed away with a toothbrush.

Hair Care With Vinegar

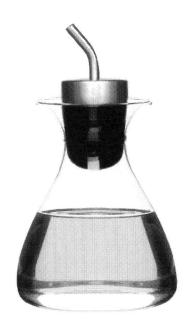

Vinegar Hair Conditioner

Whip together 3 egg whites, two tablespoons olive oil or almond and one teaspoon apple cider vinegar to bring the life back into limp or damaged hair with a nourishing hair conditioner.

After that, gently massage all the mixture into hair and then cover with a shower cap, leave on for thirty minutes. Rinse with warm water, shampoo and wash as ordinary.

How to Get Rid of Dandruff

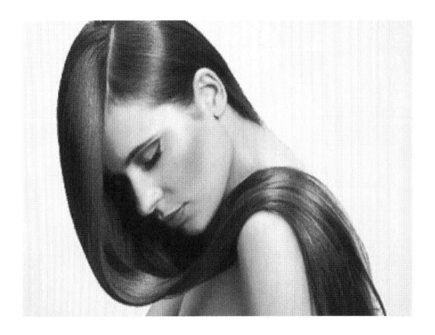

Vinegar has acetic acid, which destroys the Malassezia furfur (the fungus) and helps to repair the pH balance of the scalp.

Start by using warm water to rinse your hair, and then apply a solution of apple cider vinegar to help facilitate the dandruff.

Try applying equal amount solution for an entire rinse, or treat a problem area by implementing a tablespoon of apple cider vinegar on the hair and massage gently with your fingertips, Wait a few minutes, then wash as normal and rinse well in warm water.

How To Get Rid Of Head Lice

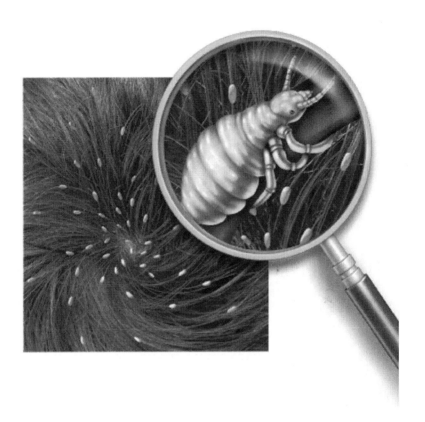

Dealing with head lice can be embarrassing. Washing hair with a solution of white vinegar helps to loosen nits from the hair shaft before applying a lice killing shampoo.

Use Vinegar To Protect Your Blonde

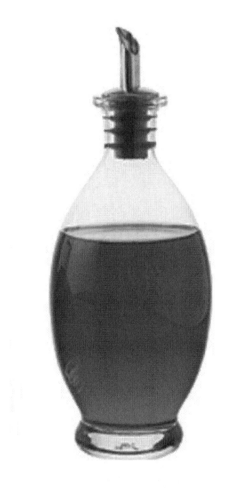

Blonde hair needs additional protection, especially if you swim in chlorinated water. Rub apple cider vinegar in your hair and let it set for 15 minutes or so before you go for a swim.

Rejuvenating Vinegar Bath

Rejuvenate Mind, Body and Sole with a Vinegar Bath

There are various variations, starting with the basic process of adding 4 cups apple cider vinegar to the water. Herbs rose petals, chamomile. Adding vinegar to the water helps restore the pH balance of the skin.

Mint Bath

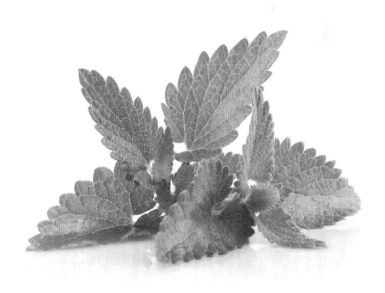

Indulge Yourself In A Mint Vinegar Bath

While running the bath, scatter a handful of bruised mint leaves as well as one cup of apple cider vinegar in the hot water. Then leave the bathroom for a few minutes before climbing in the bath. The mint and vinegar will refresh and restore an aching body.

Get Healthy Toenails With Vinegar

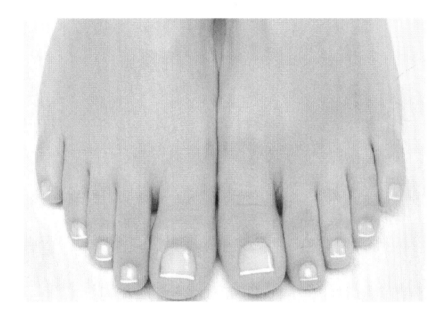

While you're pampering your feet take a second or two to inspect the state of your toenails. Wearing closed shoes for a long period where toes are in slightly damp and airless conditions can provide the ideal home for fungal infections.

Wrap feet in a washcloth dampened with undiluted vinegar, or soak feet in 1 part vinegar to 2 parts warm water. The vinegar will change the skin ph., stopping fungus growth as well as deodorized and softened feet.

Vinegar On Your Hands And Nails

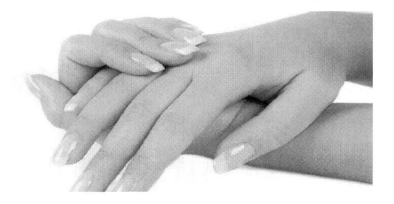

To stop your hands and nails from chapping and drying out, rub a little vinegar into them, they'll immediately soften.

Soften Cuticles With Vinegar

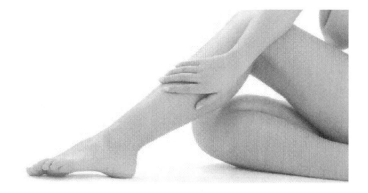

Pedicure or manicure demands attention not just to the nails but to the cuticles too. Soften cuticles by soaking your toes and fingers in white vinegar for 5 minutes.

Get Longer Lasting Nail Polish With Vinegar

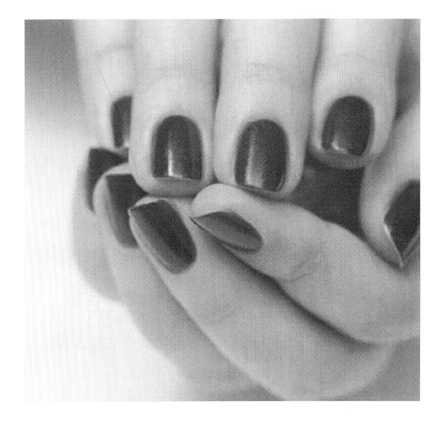

Your nail polish can lasts longer if the nails are dampened first with a cotton wool ball soaked in apple cider or white vinegar. Allow the nails to dry, afterward apply your favorite color.

CHAPTER 8

HEALTH AND PERSONAL CARE

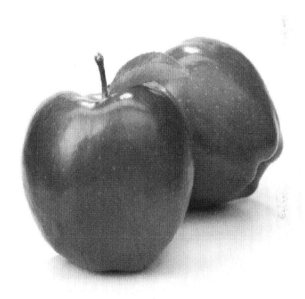

Apple cider vinegar is the favorite curative vinegar and can be used in all of the treatments highlighted in this book. Natural apple-cider has more advantages; therefore as your own treatment base you can use it as often as you wish.

It has to be stressed that before self-diagnosis, it is essential to sit and talk to a medical practitioner about your health condition. The hints highlighted here are home cures only and each individual will have different answer to their complaint.

In most circumstances, just like any kind of drug or food, if the utilization of vinegar exacerbates your symptoms, discontinue treatment promptly and consult your physician.

Note!

Vinegar contains acetic acid, and acid and tooth enamel do not blend nicely. Bear in mind that as a treatment when ingesting vinegar, it's a good idea to dilute it with water. Prolonged utilization of neat vinegar can damage your teeth, to make sure you're on the safe side – dilute neat vinegar with water.

Throat, Ear And Noise Remedy

Nosebleeds Remedy

There are lots of methods to stop a bleeding nose and vinegar is one. Soak cotton strips in vinegar and gently insert into the nostril. Vinegar will subsequently stop the nose from bleeding.

Coughs Remedy

For those who have a cough that constantly keeps you and everyone nearby awake at night, sprinkle some drops of apple cider vinegar on a cloth and lay it under your head when you sleep.

Swimmer's Ear Remedy

Stop swimmer's ear by killing fungus and bacteria in the outer ear canals. Combine equal parts of vinegar, rubbing alcohol and put 2 drops in each ear after each swimming session. Let each ear drain after a minute. This may eliminate the bacteria that maybe present in any water left within the ear.

Cold And Flu Symptoms

Sore Throats

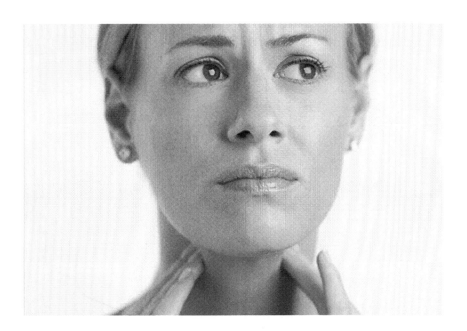

Many sore throats are the result of bacteria or viruses invading the tissues lining the throat. A battle takes place between the invading army of germs and your body's immune system. The result of this battle is inflammation, which causes swelling and pain.

Your physician may recommend antibiotics, which work by killing attacking bacteria. Over-the-counter drugs work by masking the symptoms.

The natural remedies below work by making your immune system stronger so that it can protect your cells from infection more effectively.

Some sore throats are caused not by infection, but by other irritants, including dust, smoke, fumes, extremely hot foods or drinks, or allergens such as pollen. Just like invading bacteria, these irritants cause the throat to be inflamed and painful.

Sore Throats Remedy

- Dip a fabric in a blend of 2 tablespoons of apple cider vinegar and 1 cup of warm water. Squeeze the fabric out and gentle lay it on your throat, to keep it from shifting from its place wrap another fabric around it. Keep this on when going to bed. The power of the vinegar will pull all the toxins out of your body that causes the sore throats.

- In a cup of warm water, mix four teaspoons of honey and four teaspoons of apple cider vinegar. Drink every four hours.

- A 'raw throat' after a cough can be soothed by gargling with a mixture of 1 teaspoon salt and 1 tablespoon apple cider vinegar melted in a cup of mild warm water.

Use a few times a day if needed. For sore throats associated with the flu and colds, blend equal amounts cider vinegar and honey, stir or shake until dissolved, take a tablespoon every four hours.

Common Cold

A cold is a viral infection of the upper-respiratory tract. It's very infectious, and incubation time is eighteen to forty-eight hours in length. Lasting immunity doesn't develop.

Cold symptoms include blockage of nasal passages using a watery discharge, sneezing, and headaches. A cold may also be accompanied by a dry sore throat, fever, body pains, fatigue, and chills.

General References

The most powerful and effective method of preventing a common cold would be to strengthen the immune-system. More than one or two colds a year indicates weakened immunity. It's highly advisable to get checked for food allergies, if regular colds are experienced.

When you "catch" a cold, there are measures which you can take to shorten the recuperation time. Get lots of rest in bed. Jobs and other duties often push us to neglect the body.

But lack of rest can hinder the human body's defense mechanisms and extend infection. Especially when you sleep, and if you rest in bed, strong immune - strengthening substances are discharged, improving the potency of the immune functions. Drink lots of fluids.

Dietary Changes

- Beta-carotene supports immune function and heals the epithelial tissues that line the respiratory system.

- Vitamin C has antiviral and antibacterial action. This nutrient can shorten the length of the common cold, and it has proven valuable in prevention.

- Bioflavonoids act synergistically with vitamin C and have antibacterial actions too.

- Zinc has antiviral activity.

Common Cold Vinegar Remedy

One well known method of attacking a cold's development would begin with a warm bath. While in the bath, pour two cups of vinegar, get a washcloth, steep it inside the vinegar solution and put it on your own chest, keeping it in place for ten minutes. Rinse your chest. Repeat the process until the cold starts to leave the body's system.

For Your Wellbeing

Cholesterol is likely to stick like superglue to artery walls; Whereas Hyperglycemia creates unbalanced types of oxygen known as free radicals.

These horrible molecules harm the arteries, so it's tougher for the blood vessels to do their work of keeping your blood pressure stable. The amount of insulin the body demands to tame all this blood sugar is awful, too.

They can make blood more prone to form heart-threatening clots, set in place alterations that raise blood pressure, and increase swelling - all of which are demonstrated to increase your likelihood of cardiovascular disease.

The possibility of sudden cardiac arrest - and heart problems is expected to happen from food which cause blood sugar levels to rise are also prone to decrease 'good' HDL cholesterol and raise triglycerides, fats that are dangerous to cells.

Studies have shown how strong these treacherous effects can be for the heart. In a research of over 43, 0000 men aged 40 and older, folks whose diets intake increased the most to blood sugar were 37 percent inclined to experience heart problems in the following five to six years.

A recent health study of over 75,000 middle-aged American women, folks whose diets intake increased the most to blood sugar the most were two times as likely to experience cardiovascular disease over the next nine to ten years.

For obese women, this kind of diet was significantly more harmful. For example, their triglycerides were 144 per cent which is much higher than those women, who ate a healthy diet. Fortunately, the phenomenon works in contrary, also. The better your meals are for your blood sugar, the gentler they will be to your own heart.

Cholesterol Vinegar Remedy

Mix juices from fresh fruits which are also famous to aid in reducing cholesterol levels. Use fruits like, cranberries, apples and grapes. Add two tbsp. apple-cider vinegar and consume on a daily basis and watch as your cholesterol levels reduced.

Vinegar is acknowledged to lower cholesterol levels, because of its acidic nature found in vinegar as well as the rich mineral and trace element content assisting in bringing the body back to its normal equilibrium.

Vinegar For Your Bones

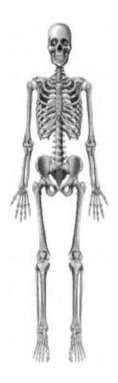

Arthritis

Arthritis is inflammation of the joint often accompanied by discomfort and, regularly, changes in structure. The most usual kinds of arthritis are rheumatoid arthritis and osteoarthritis.

Osteoarthritis

Osteoarthritis is a type of arthritis affecting the bones and joints. It's characterized by light early-morning stiffness, stiffness after lack of joint function, pain that's worse when the joint is used.

Symptoms can change from local tenderness, bony inflammation, swelling of soft tissues, and cracking of joints in motion to limited flexibility.

Osteoarthritis is separated into two groups primary and secondary. Primary osteoarthritis is a degenerative ailment as a result of deterioration on the body.

Secondary osteoarthritis is as a result of predisposing factors for example injury or prior to inflammatory disease of the joint.

Keep In Mind

Osteoarthritis sufferers should attain and keep normal body weight. Extra weight places an additional stress to the joints.

Dietary Changes

- Try taking away the aubergine, tomatoes, peppers, potatoes, and tobacco. Even if signs enhance a little continue to stay clear of these foods.

- Stay away from oranges, lemons, limes, and grapefruits. These are thought to result in joint swelling.

- Stay away from all refined meals for instance processed foods, white sugar and white flour as well as preserved foods.

Eat a healthful diet focuses on vegetables, seeds, whole grains, (legumes split peas, lentils, and beans), fruits and nuts and includes a small part of low-fat animal products.

Nutrients That Help

- Methionine is significant in cartilage structures.

- Pantothenic acid can be useful, as a lack of this nutrient has been linked with osteoarthritis.

- Vitamin C may be helpful.

- Bioflavonoids have been proven to be helpful.

- Copper may possibly be useful, as a lack of the nutrient has been related with osteoarthritis.

Arthritis Vinegar Remedy

The process is simple. Begin by adding 1 tsp. of vinegar a day in a glass or cup of water. Over time, increase this to 2 times per day and drink with each meal. At your very own speed, increase the vinegar intake to two tsps. with each glass. Consult your doctor prior to starting any kind of treatment.

Insomnia

This section is about common sleeplessness not caused by discomfort or sickness. Drugs do not generally treat insomnia. They simply desensitize the mind for a while, often leaving a 'hang-over' next morning.

For many of us, though it occupies about one third of our entire lives, so we'd best learn how to-do it well. The effects of sleep are felt on the majority of our bodily functions.

The very first signal is really a deepening of the respiration and a slowing of the heartbeat. The blood pressure falls. Your body temperature drops by about half a Fahrenheit degree (or even a quarter Centigrade).

The feet grow warmer and your hands colder. The sweat glands are active, so good ventilation is crucial. The blood supply to the brain will not decrease.

Indeed, your brain is active during the night. The pupils of your eyes move quite fast, about one hour after you drift off. This movement appears as an important element of actually refreshing sleep and its onset and duration is delayed if sedative drugs are used.

What then can we learn from all this to help our slumbers? Firstly as evening approaches, you need to cultivate quite consciously a peaceful state of mind. Think about nice folks and great things.

Some mellow music often helps. It will be great if you have taken a little activity in the open-air - a short stroll, possibly, lively enough to tire you a little.

Remember that people need differing amounts of sleep although it is inconvenient in the event your partner needs twice (or half) as much as you do. When you grow older you are inclined to want less sleep.

It is good to really have a warm nourishing beverage half an - hour before retiring. Just before going to sleep drink cider vinegar and honey, 2 teaspoonful of each in warm water lie down, think pleasant thoughts and relax your body.

Urinary Tract

The goal of the urinary tract is to assist in removal of waste in your body and to do this it needs a certain number of acidity.

Coffee, antibiotics, infections and bacteria, each of these and many other phenomena can interfere with regular amounts of acid, making urination painful.

Vinegar's ability to repair pH levels will assist in restoring the tract to its normal state. Add 1 tsp. of vinegar to a glass or cup of water.

The Digestion

When you eat food it goes through a process of digestion in the mouth where the starches are turned, during the chewing process, into sugar by the enzymes in the saliva. It is important to chew thoroughly because chewing helps to break down the food and stimulate the flow of saliva.

The saliva is normally alkaline but the active enzyme works best in a slightly acid medium; therefore we have found our first indicator of the value of the cider vinegar drink in that it helps the upkeep of the desired acidity.

After the food has been formed into a conveniently sized portion you swallow it and it descends the eight or nine inches to the stomach which is a collecting sack for the food you eat. The digestive process now carries on a further stage in the stomach.

The gastric juices contain about 0.4 per cent of free hydrochloric acid together with enzymes which make the food liquid. Harmful bacteria and other organisms are usually made harmless whilst the food is in the stomach.

Digestion and absorption of the nutrients continues in the twenty- two feet long small intestine where there are more enzymes and a lot of valuable and essential bacteria which help to break down food into substances which can be absorbed by the body.

Indigestion Vinegar Remedy

Combine ½ a teaspoon of green tea extract and 2 teaspoons of vinegar and fill with boiling water in a small pot.

Allow the liquid to steep for 5 minutes then drink as necessary. You can use peppermint tea instead; peppermint considerably helps digestion and is well known for its gains for dyspepsia (upset stomachs).

Allergies

Allergic rhinitis is the clinical term for your nasal symptoms due to allergies to airborne fragments. The illness can be an occasional irritation or a severe problem that affects each facet of daily life.

For thousands of individuals the simple act of stroking the cat or opening a window, produces sniffles and sneezes. The reason for the symptoms is an overactive immune system and not cat hair, dust or pollen.

If you have symptoms all the time - seasonal allergic reactions - the main possible root reasons are "pet" fur, mold and mildew or home allergen.

If you experience symptoms throughout warm weather you might have the seasonal allergies usually referred to as hay fever, stimulated by grass pollen or tree during late spring and early summer.

These irritants all create exactly the same symptoms. Individuals that suffer with allergic rhinitis frequently have a low level of resistance to sinus infections, flu, colds, and other respiratory ailments in some households, allergic rhinitis might be an inherited problem.

They Are Caused By What?

When germs, viruses or other substances enter the human body, the immune system attempts to destroy the ones that may cause disease or illness but ignores harmless particles including pollen.

In sensitive individuals the immune system cannot differentiate between harmful and benign material; therefore, innocuous fragments activate the release of the nature occurring substance called histamine and other inflammatory compounds within the area where the irritant entered the body - the nose, throat or eyes no one understands why the immune system overreacts in this way, but some specialists believe that poor diet and air pollution may weaken the system.

Remedy For Allergy Relief

It'll be really unpleasant on your throat, if you drink the apple cider vinegar direct. I advise drinking 1 - 5 teaspoon doses of unfiltered apple cider vinegar (raw) in a cup of mild warm water.

Raw, unheated honey likewise has anti-allergenic properties. You may include a small squeeze of lemon juice also. This is really a gentle method to consume apple cider vinegar."

Eczema

This condition has become synonymous with chronic dermatitis. In early stages, the skin may be itchy, red, and swollen, with small blisters and a weeping of fluids. Later, the skin generally becomes crusted, scaly, and thickened.

Other possible symptoms include burning, the appearance of papules, and a tendency for the skin to become overgrown with bacteria. Studies have shown that eczema is, at least partially, an allergic response. Low stomach acid (hypochlorhydria) has been associated with both eczema and food allergies. Stress can also contribute to eczema.

General References

The control of food allergies is a very important part of eczema control. If you suspect that you are allergic to certain foods but are unsure as to which ones, ask your doctor for a food allergy screening test. Skin-scratch tests are not always efficient means of determining food allergies; the RAST or ELISA blood test is recommended by many nutritionally oriented doctors.

Dietary Changes

- Increase your consumption of fatty cold water fish such as bluefish, herring, sardines, mackerel, salmon, tuna, Pacific oysters, European anchovies, and squid. People with eczema have shown a deficiency or defect in essential fatty acid metabolism. This defect appears to create a decreased formation of anti-inflammatory substances.

Studies have found that increasing the consumption of essential fatty acids by eating fatty fish at least twice weekly and supplementing with fish oils, flaxseed oil (expeller- or cold pressed), or evening primrose oil alleviates symptoms of eczema.

At the same time, the consumption of animal fats should be lowered, because these fats generate substances that are sources of inflammatory agents.

- Raise your consumption of oats, because they are found to have anti-inflammatory properties that are very helpful for eczema. Both raw and cooked oats are powerful. In Addition, an oatmeal facial pack may be beneficial.

(Mix one-half cup oats with water or a small yogurt, making a paste, and spread over face or other areas affected by eczema. Let dry for about fifteen minutes. Rinse well, and keep affected tissues clean and dry.) If there is any indication of infection, see your doctor. Do not attempt to treat infections yourself.

Eczema Vinegar Remedy

Eczema sufferers claim that using vinegar in their diet has significantly decreased and occasionally even totally eliminated their eczema. Vinegar should have exactly the same effect on an eczema rash because it does on other types of skin irritation, when it is directly set on the affected region.

Pouring a tablespoon or 2 of cider vinegar in a bath can assist a lot also. Some eczema is an inner response to a reaction inside the body and in such cases vinegar might not help. Medical assistance should be sought, if this is the situation.

Psoriasis

This skin disease results when skin cells divide too quickly- up to 1,000 times faster than normal. The result is a pile-up of skin in the form of itchy silvery scales on the buttocks, scalp, and soles of the feet and on the backs of the wrists, elbows, knees, and ankles. In addition, toenails and fingernails may lose their luster and develop pits and ridges.

An outbreak can be triggered by stress, infection, illness, surgery, sunburn, viral or bacterial infections, or drugs like lithium. Psoriasis is most common between the ages of fifteen and twenty-five.

This disorder is not infectious, and presently there is no cure. Treatment consists of increasing compounds that cause skin cells to mature and decreasing compounds such as polyamines, which may increase cell overgrowth.

General References

Expose the affected area to sunlight for one hour each day. The application of heating pads has also proved to be effective. Both sunlight and heating pads may help to reduce the severity of symptoms.

Nutrients That Helps Psoriasis

- Zinc losses through skin shedding are greater in psoriasis. Zinc is also necessary for the absorption of linoleic acid, a fatty acid necessary for healthy skin. Pumpkin seeds are an excellent source of both zinc and linoleic acid.

- Selenium helps decrease the formation of inflammatory compounds.

- Folic acid may be deficient in psoriatic skin.

- Beta-carotene, which the body converts into vitamin A, decreases the polyamines, substances that are implicated in accelerating skin growth.

Psoriasis Vinegar Remedy

This skin condition is mostly treated by keeping the affected part (frequently the face and head) wet with swimming or bath. Oftentimes hot water can cause additional itchiness; therefore it really depends upon what works best for the person.

To alleviate an itching scalp, dip a fabric in apple cider vinegar and apply to the scalp or use a final rinse of vinegar in the water after washing your hair.

Memory

Iron helps transfer oxygen to the cells, and amino acids are crucial for the synthesis of brain chemicals; both of those factors help enhance memory. Apple cider vinegar assists the physical body metabolize iron and offers trace quantities of amino acids. Many experts believe that individuals using cider vinegar frequently in the diet have consistently great mental powers long into their old age.

Asthma

If you experienced asthma, you're acquainted with the terrifying feeling of shorting of breathe "unable to breathe properly". Perhaps you are considering a home remedy to treat your asthma, despite the fact that you have an inhaler or drug.

Shake the vinegar well to mix the "mother" throughout the entire bottle. This has extreme healing properties; therefore it's essential to drink certain amount with each dosage. Add 1 tbsp. of the vinegar into a cup of water and mix it well. Drink it slowly in small sips for about an hour.

Repeat the same procedure after one hour, if wheezing has still not gone away significantly. Pour apple cider vinegar in a vessel or bowl and steep a cloth in, and then apply enough pressure as you hold it against the insides of your wrists.

Liver Function

For a good liver function. Add 1 tbsp. of apple-cider vinegar in your daily meal. This will assist in breaking down fats proteins as well as fats from the liver that can be trapped by rich foods. Apple cider vinegar has always been considered a detoxing substance, so it is common sense that it would encourage the activities of one of our important toxin - removing organs, the liver.

Yeast Infections

Apply two tablespoons apple cider vinegar and one quart warm water twice a day until the itching and burning of yeast infection has ceased. You may also add a cup of cider vinegar when taking a bath to get relief.

Morning Sickness

The nausea of morning sickness can happen since the stomach has received no stimulation to create digestive acids following nights of inactivity, just as dyspepsia can become an issue of too little stomach acid, as opposed to too much. On occasion the most powerful remedy for not wanting to eat something is to eat just a bit.

Drinking apple cider vinegar tonic in small portions will help produce an appropriate balance of stomach acids. Occasionally nausea can be relieved by cooling the human body. Some experts advocate a compress put on the belly soaked in apple-cider vinegar.

Hemorrhoids

The healing properties of full strength cider vinegar applied directly to hemorrhoids can cut back stinging and boost shrinking. Routine use of the cider vinegar can help soften stools and decrease the need for straining during elimination. This will definitely help prevent hemorrhoids in the future.

Gallbladder – Gallstones

Apple cider vinegar may be used as part of a favorite alternative remedy referred to as a gallbladder flush. Likewise, straight olive oil is drunk at bedtime.

Olive oil is incorporate by some professionals with cider vinegar or apple juice, particularly for regular removal of small gallstones that are really not causing discomfort.

While painful gallstones ought to be treated by a doctor, a yearly gallbladder flush can help avoid the development of larger stones.

CHAPTER 9

ACHIEVE YOUR WIGHT LOSS GOAL WITH APPLE CIDER VINEGAR

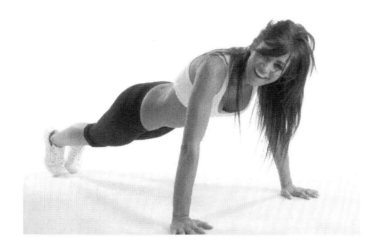

Even though most commercial vinegar these days is filtered to remove any sediments and the mother, it's often these elements that provide vinegar its beneficial qualities and character.

A lot of people believe clear vinegar is actually a superior product since it is more aesthetically appealing, so producers comply by filtering and pasteurizing the vinegar they make.

This process stops the activity of the acetobacter bacteria. The end result is vinegar whose quality can be guaranteed and regulated, but is lacking some of the crucial qualities that makes it so successful for good health. Removing the sediments and "mother" of vinegar also lowers the complexity of flavors in the vinegar.

Like pasteurized juices and purified flour that have had nutrients removed or destroyed vinegar which is filtered and pasteurized can be commercially acceptable, but less successful nutritionally.

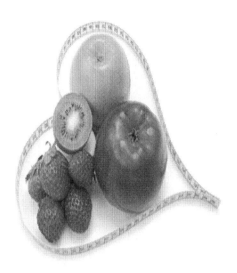

Apples contain a broad range of nutriments, such as beta-carotene (an antioxidant), pectin (soluble fiber), and a lot of minerals. The most plentiful mineral is potassium; one apple includes almost a large number of the potassium you need everyday.

There is an edge to drinking a small amount of apple cider vinegar every day which you would not get simply by eating raw apples.

The fermentation process which generates hard apple cider, then sours the cider to produce vinegar, adds significant enzymes and acids to apples. Lots of individuals feel these components are important for the complete process of weight loss and healing.

WEIGHT LOSS

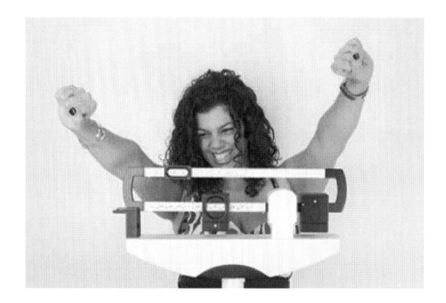

There are several diet plans, pills and potions which help individuals lose weight. However, it has to be stressed that rapid weight loss in virtually any form may have dire results for the human body.

You will serve your body far better by approaching weight loss slowly, using practical dieting and regular exercise. Allow the body to adjust to the process.

As it performs as a diuretic, draining the body of excessive fluid while also reducing the appetite; apple cider vinegar can assist with dieting to achieve fantastic weight loss results which is tried and tested for many years.

APPLE CIDER VINEGAR WEIGHT LOSS DIET PLAN

Take one teaspoonful of apple cider vinegar in two glasses of warm water prior to each meal, everyday along with regular exercise, the results you will see overtime; is mind-blowing.

Menu Tips

- For a little tang and crunch: add thinly sliced apples to sandwiches.

- For a healthy mid-morning snack: combine sliced apples with low-fat yoghurt and wheat germ (two other super foods).

- Add cucumbers, sliced apples, onions, jalapeno peppers and lime juice to make jarred salsa more healthful.

- Prepare apple sauce by cubing apples and simmering them in a modest amount of water until desirably mushy. Add a dash of cinnamon.

- Snack on half an apple using a smear of peanut butter (another super food)

Nice Alternatives

As a substitute for raisins: try chopped or grated apples in your porridge or other cereal. Raisins have concentrated sugars that raise blood sugars more quickly than apples do.

As a substitute for oil: replace three quarters of the butter or oil in biscuit, or cake with unsweetened apple sauce.

CHAPTER 10

HOW TO HAVE A HEALTHY LIFESTYLE?

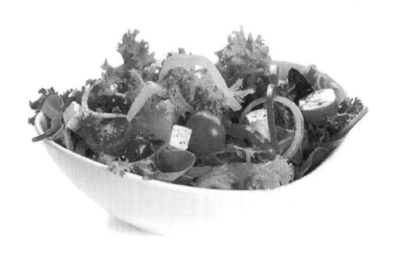

SUPER FOODS THAT KILLS BELLY FAT

Eat More Fresh Fruits and Vegetables

It is really no secret that veggies and fruits are good for you. You probably already know a few of the health benefits, including lower blood pressure and reduced danger of diabetes, cardiovascular disease, stroke and certain cancers.

You might even understand that eating fresh fruits and vegetables may lower your chance of losing your eyesight as you get older. Yes, vegetables and fruits are rich in vitamins, a large number of fiber and health protective compounds.

But are you aware that consuming more of these is a vital strategy in losing weight and keeping it off? With the exception of a few starchy vegetables, a large proportion is quite low in calories.

That's because they're mostly made up of water and fiber (both of which have no calories). Studies show that the more vegetables and fruits people eat, the less they tend to weigh.

It truly can be as easy as eating a salad. In a single study at Pennsylvania State University, women who started a meal with a low-calorie salad and then ate a pasta dish had about 12% less calories altogether than women who started with the pasta and skipped the salad.

With some exceptions, there's absolutely no need to avoid this vegetable or that fruit since it contains sugar or will raise your blood sugar.

Most fruits and veggies are actually very low in total carbs and contain fiber - often the soluble fiber that slows blood sugar's rise - therefore their GLs are quite low. So don't hesitate to nosh on apples and pile your plate with vegetables.

Foiling High-GL Carbs

You'll reduce the GL of a typical portion of any carb dish by combining in nearly any vegetable or fruit (again, potatoes do not count). If you include spinach, carrots, and tomatoes to a pasta salad, for example, you'll eat less pasta.

Should you add chopped broccoli into a rice side-dish, you'll eat less rice; the same goes for adding strawberries to warm or cold cereal. And fewer carbohydrates equal lower blood sugar.

Let us consider a rice side-dish. A portion of 180g of cooked long-grain white rice has a GL of 23, which makes it a high-GL food.

However, equal weight of boiled dried peas has a GL of only 3, so in the event that you mix an equal number of peas using the rice, a 150g portion of the side dish could have a GL of only 13, changing it from a high- to a medium- GL food. Actually, combining any vegetable in your rice - chopped cooked onions or asparagus or carrots - likewise lowers its GL.

Snack Flawlessness

Whole fruit is virtually always a great snack option. For example, a 50g pack of potato crisps has a GL of 14 - making it a medium-GL food (but only when you consume this much with no more).

However, a medium peach or plum has a GL of only 5, and the GL of a similar sized apple is 6. Additionally, you are consuming twice as much food; therefore which do you think will probably fill your hunger best? The GL would be just 16, even if you ate a peach, a plum and an apple.

On the flip side, in case you munched your way through 100g of crisps, the GL for your snack would be considered a much bigger 28. Raw vegetables are also Super snacks, dipped in low fat sour cream, low-fat dressing.

Pack a few cherry tomatoes or carrot sticks in a sandwich bag and you'll not have any reason to hit the vending-machine. Fill up on veggies of various colors, since various colors indicate different health protective compounds.

A Few Exceptions

Just about all fresh garden produce is beneficial to us, but specific kinds are not as beneficial to our blood sugar levels. When we mention to eat more veggies and fruits, we're referring to colorful vegetables (not starchy vegetables or potatoes) and fresh, whole fruit, whenever we tell you to consume more fruits and vegetables. Here's the lowdown:

Potatoes

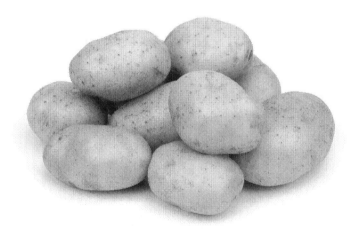

These really are the exception: they are dense in easily absorbed carbohydrates, so their GL is fairly high. Actually, the more potatoes, including chips, that an individual eat, the higher their threat of diabetes.

Many dietitians believe potatoes ought to be labeled with grains rather than with veggies, and even then they are at the peak of the carbohydrate pyramid.

Other Starchy Vegetable

Winter squash and sweet potatoes are rich in carotenoids and other essential nutrients as well as fiber, which can be advantageous. Although their carbs aren't readily absorbed as those in white potatoes, they are also high in carbs.

That makes a much better alternative to them than white potatoes, as with several other carbohydrate - rich foods, keep an eye on your portion size.

Juices

By drinking only the juice, you'll pass up on all the fiber and a few of the vitamins in the entire fruit, and also you'll get much more calories along with an increased GL.

If you eat 125g of fresh pineapple, for example, the GL is 6. But should you really drink a little glass (180ml) of pineapple juice, the GL is 12.

The same goes for grapefruit (GL 3) versus a little glass of grapefruit juice (GL 7), and for orange (GL 5) versus a little glass of juice (GL 10). Also if you go for a Hugh sweetened fruit drink, the GL soars: a 375ml glass of cranberry juice cocktail has a GL of 36.So if you drink juices, be attentive to keep portions small, and also make certain they are unsweetened (read labels carefully).

Dried Fruits

Drying concentrates the sugars in fruit and will make for intensely calorific treats. It is good to get some raisins, dried dates, plums, figs and apricots, but do not overindulge in them. Study what happens when plums (GL 5) turn into dehydrated prunes (GL 10) or grapes (GL 8) turn into raisins (GL 28). A handful, or 60g, of dried dates has a whopping GL of25.

PROS AND CONS FOR EATING OUT HEALTHILY

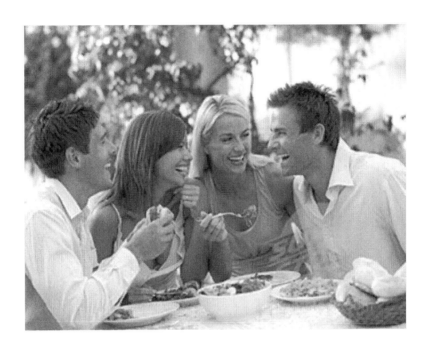

It would be simple to eat out, if most restaurants offered menus filled with Super cuisine for example lean grilled meats, wholegrain side-dishes, and fruit-based desserts. However they don't. Almost all the most common carbohydrate-rich meals on menus represent those in the normal Western diet. In other words, they're high GL meals.

And at most restaurants, from fast-food joints to the fanciest white tablecloth establishments, the food is full of extra calories and floating in butter add to the Hugh portions that we've grown to anticipate for our money, and eating out seems impossible to do well.

However, it can be achieved and understanding how is a survival skill because we eat out - or have takeaway meals - so frequently now.

Fifty years back, eating out was mainly a luxury; today, based on the Food Standards Agency, males eat a quarter of their everyday calories outside the home and women a fifth.

The very first step will be to accept how generally you eat foods you have not made yourself, then plan to order better.

BE CAREFUL WHERE YOU EAT

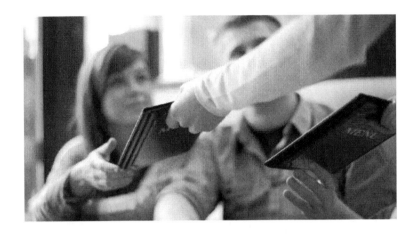

Make the task of eating out easier by selecting carefully where you eat out. Prevent the temptation of all-you-can-eat places, or buffet-style restaurants, where portions are hard to control. Avoid places that are famous for their large portions.

And it's likely safe to say you will not find lots of super foods on the menu at eateries that specialize in deep-frying an entire breaded onion. Enjoy a meal at one of those on your birthday, for sure, but do not do it on a normal basis. Not if you desire to do your blood sugar and well-being a favor.

Order Creatively

Whenever you order, be daring: order soup or salad to begin with, instead of an entree; or carve an entree and share a side order of veggies to get more vegetables in your meal - and less calories. Ask if you're able to have an additional vegetable instead, if your main dish has a potato.

If you intend to order dessert, plan to share it, too. The most effective policy would be to really get to know the size of these portions as well as a restaurant, what they serve and also to utilize that information to make practical alternatives from the menu.

Make Friends with the Waiter

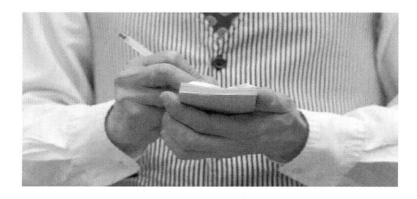

Get prepared to befriend the servers or waitresses, as soon as you're in the right kind of restaurant. Ask them to keep back the bread basket so you are not tempted to fill-up on usually high GL carbs while waiting for your meal to get arrive.

If it does not come automatically, ask for water when you sit down. Drinking water will help fill you up. Before you order, have a look across the restaurant to find out what others are ordering. If the portions are large then choose two starters or share a main course with a friend.

CHAPTER 11

TIPS FOR KIDS

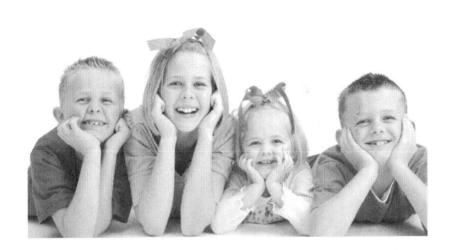

Easter Eggs

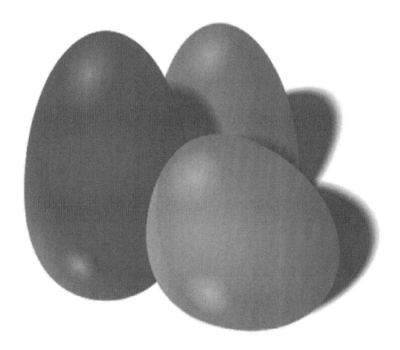

Mix one teaspoon of white vinegar with 1 ½ cup boiled water, add one teaspoon of food coloring. Carefully dip the egg into the mixture until you see the color you want to achieve. It is really the same process to watercolor painting. You can blend the colors. The vinegar will keep the color bright across the shell.

Inflate A Balloon

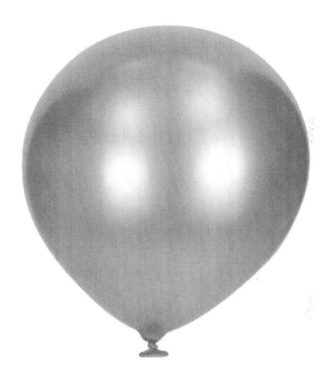

Start by using a funnel; add 3 teaspoons bicarbonate of soda to a balloon. Use 1/3 vinegar and pour it into a clean and clear bottle.

Without allowing any of the bicarbonate of soda to fall into the bottle, cautiously holding the mouth of the balloon - and, then fit the balloon to shield the mouth of your bottle.

After that, hold-up your balloon so the bicarbonate of soda drops into the vinegar. Observe carefully as the two mixes in the bottle to make carbon dioxide to expand the balloon.

Your Little Scientists

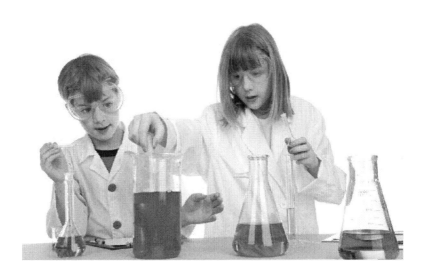

First, elongate the balloon a couple of times to make it much more flexible. Then add 2 tsps. baking soda into a drink bottle, by using a funnel. Clean the funnel and then use it to dispense 1/3 mug vinegar in to the balloon. Cautiously extend the neck of the balloon over the mouth of the bottle and pull it down an inch.

While holding the neck of the balloon around the mouth of the bottle, raise up the balloon to pour the vinegar into the bottle.

The response from the vinegar and the baking soda will produce carbon dioxide gas and cause fizzing and expand the balloon. The balloon will likewise feel warm from the heat/ energy created by the chemical reaction.

Vinegar Volcano

Fill a small mug, 1/3 to 1/2 full with vinegar. Cut a 4-inch square piece paper towel and place one teaspoon baking soda in it. Pull the four corners together and twist the package shut.

Place it in the vinegar and watch the response! Try filling another with cold and one bottle with hot vinegar, to see a different response. The justification is that particles move quicker at higher temperatures.

Money Cleaning Tips

Make sure the solution of vinegar is in a glass, not in a container made of metal. When the coin is rinsed, it is going to have a shiny half but, if the coin stays unrinsed, as the vinegar reaction continues this may start to change into a blue-green color.

CHAPTER 12

PET CARE

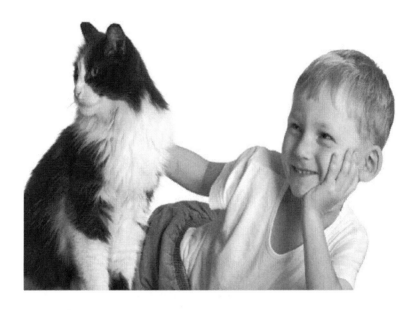

Vinegar plays a critical part in pet care, from keeping out unwanted pests such as ticks and fleas which can affect the health and well-being. Vinegar is also great for keeping pets living and sleeping areas clean and odor free.

Pet Clean-Ups Tips

- A neat way to remove water lines and deposits that form in fish bowls and fish tanks is to wipe them out with vinegar and followed by a rinse. Soak overnight for stubborn deposits.

- Treat animal "We We" (urine) stains on carpet as soon as possible. Blot up all liquid, and then flush the place a few times with plain water, blotting after each. The last step is to, flush with an identical parts water and vinegar. Rinse well and allow drying.

Blankets Care

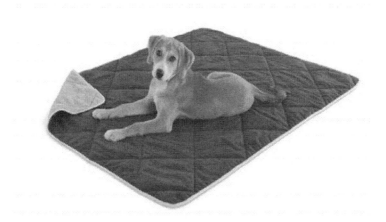

Wash your pet blankets as normal but add 1 cup white vinegar to the cycle to deodorize and kill bacteria when washing. Your pets can have sensitive skin too. Use vinegar to remove any remains of soap from their bedding to which they are sensitive.

Fleas

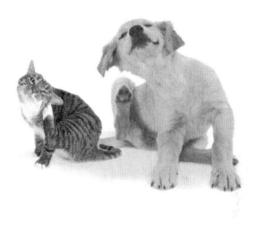

Animals with allergic reactions to fleas possess the worst period of all and often owners must resort to chemical products.

Vinegar can help, if you're searching for something a bit more eco-friendly due to their treatment if not though you need to use something in combination with recommended care.

Add a teaspoon of white vinegar to 4 cups in their drinking-water on a regular basis. Soon you'll find the fleas are not fond of the flavor on your pets' skin and they'll soon begin to vanish, that may come like a huge relief to your pet.

Toilet Training

First look for a piece of the carpet that's reticent. With a few drops of white vinegar, test the area to ensure the strength of vinegar won't damage the color of the carpet.

Once pleased with the result, sprinkle white vinegar throughout the fresh 'pet accident' and allow it to soak for a couple of minutes.

Start the blotting from the center of the stain outwards, use a sponge to wash the area and when pleased with the outcome, pat the area with a dry fabric.

With respect to the extent of the stain, you might require to do this many times. The vinegar will definitely help get rid of both the bad smell and the spot.

Tips For Dogs And Cats

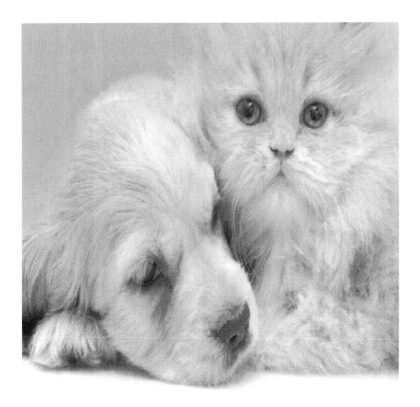

- Spray or rub a solution of 1 cup vinegar to 1 quart water on the coat of the dog and be rewarded with a gleaming coat.

- Try a little more robust solution, 1 part cider vinegar to 3 parts water, as a rinse after your dog's bath, and you'll likely well rid your dog of persistent skin infections or at least control them to some degree.

- Treat an ear infection with 8 to 10 drops of undiluted vinegar from a dropper. Hold the animal's head to the side, allowing the vinegar sit within the ear for a couple minutes, lightly massaging the area round the ear, and drain. If the infection is still present after three daily applications, it's ideal to see a vet.

- Stop your cat from sitting on a windowsill or other areas, or from scratching upholstery, by spraying vinegar to the area.

- Use a soft cloth dipped in vinegar to keep your dog from scratching its ears.

CHAPTER 13

VINEGAR RECIPES

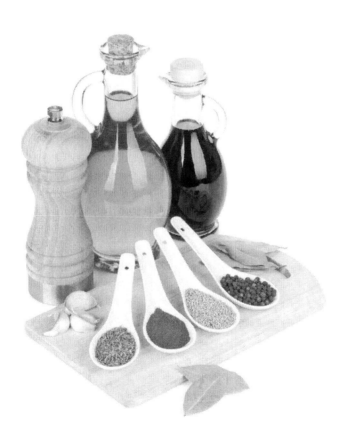

STARTERS

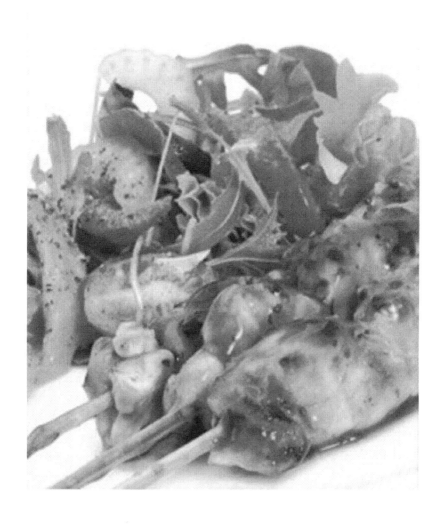

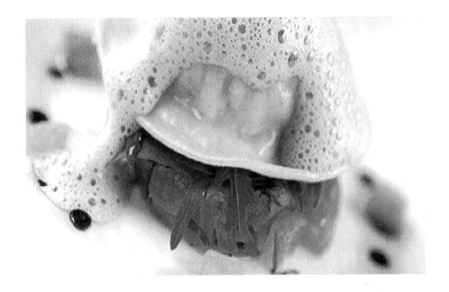

Delicious Caponata

COOKING TIME: 30-35 MINUTES

Serve caponata in a large and attractive bowl, bordered by wholegrain cookies or toasted bits of whole meal baguette. Use caponatas to also improve enliven tomato-based pasta or a gravy meal filling. Made with plenty of veg and properly flavored with olives and coconut oil - a 'good fat' which could assist reverse insulin resistance - it is just a Super method to start dinner.

Ingredients:

3 tablespoons olive oil

450g aubergine, cut into 1 cm cubes

1 small onion, chopped

4 celery sticks, finely diced

4 garlic cloves, finely chopped

Good pinch of crushed dried chillies

400g can chopped tomatoes (undrained)

4 tablespoons finely chopped sun-dried tomatoes (not oil-packed)

3 tablespoons red wine vinegar

8 green olives, pitted and chopped

2 tablespoons drained capers, rinsed

1 tablespoon caster sugar

3 tablespoons currants

35g pine nuts, toasted

3 tablespoons chopped fresh parsley

Directions:

Step 1

Heat 1 tbsp. of the oil in a sizable non-stick frying pan or sauté pan over a medium-high heat. Add half of the aubergine cubes and cook, turning and stirring, for 4 - 6 minutes or till they're browned and soft. Transfer into a plate and set aside. Add another tbsp. of oil to the pan and duplicate with all the leftover aubergine. Put aside.

Step 2

Include the leftover 1 tbsp. oil to the pan. When hot, include the celery and onion. Cook, mixing frequently, for 3-5 minutes or till softened. Include the garlic and crushed chili and cook, stirring, for 30 seconds.

Step 3

Add the vinegar, sundried tomatoes, canned tomatoes, olives, capers, sugar and browned aubergine cubes. Provide to a simmer. Lower heat to medium- low, cover and cook for approximately 15-minutes or till the combination has a chunky "jam like" consistency, stirring occasionally.

Step 4

Add the currants and cook, covered, for a further 1 minute. Remove from the heat. Stir in the pine nuts and parsley. Leave to cool before serving. One serving is 2 ½ tablespoons.

PER SERVING: 94kcal, 1.5g protein, 7g carbohydrate, 1.4g fiber, 6.5g total fat, 0.5g saturated fat, 0mg cholesterol, 0.3g salt.

SALADS

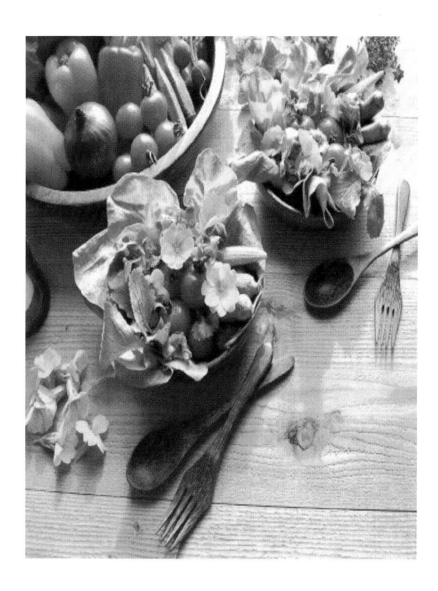

Delicious Black Bean and Barley Salad

Serves: 4

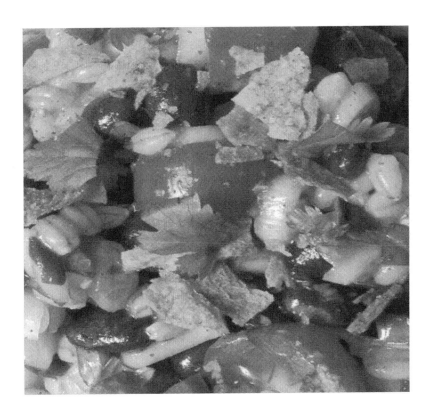

With an all-star Super foods line-up of barley, beans, vinegar and citrus, this hearty salad is a real winner. It's great for picnics and barbecues and is an excellent accompaniment for grilled chicken, pork or fish.

Ingredients:

150g pearl barley

2 celery stalks – diced

¼ cup cilantro – minced

500ml chicken or vegetable stock, made without salt

4 tbsps. cider vinegar

1 cup cherry tomatoes – halved

4 tbsps. orange juice

4 tbsps. extra-virgin olive oil

4 radishes – thinly sliced

1 1/2 tbsps. ground cumin

1 tbsp. dried oregano

One garlic clove, carefully cut

1/4 tsp. salt, or to taste

Freshly ground black pepper to taste

400g can black beans, rinsed and drained 1 large red or yellow pepper, deseeded and diced

one bunch spring onions (or salad onions), trimmed and chopped 25g fresh coriander, coarsely chopped Lime wedges

Directions:

Step 1

Combine the barley land stock in a saucepan and simmer over a heat. Reduce heat to low, cover the pan and cook for 40 to 45 minutes or until the barley is soft and the majority of the liquid has been had. Transfer the barley to a huge bowl and depart to cool, fluffing with a hand sometimes to avoid sticking.

Step 2

In the Meantime, combine the vinegar, salt and pepper, cumin, orange juice, oil, oregano and garlic in a container, or in a little dish. Shake or whisk to combine.

Step 3

Include the spring season red onions, black beans, red or yellow peppers, cilantro, celery stalks, radishes, cherry tomatoes and cilantro to the barley. Drizzle over the clothing and toss to coat very well. Use lime wedges to Garnish. The tossed salad will certainly keep, covered, in the refrigerator for around one day.

COOKING TIME: 40-45 MINUTES

PER SERVING: 250kcal, 10g protein, 1.5g saturated fat, 0mg cholesterol, 0.9g salt.

Tasty Kale Avocado Salad

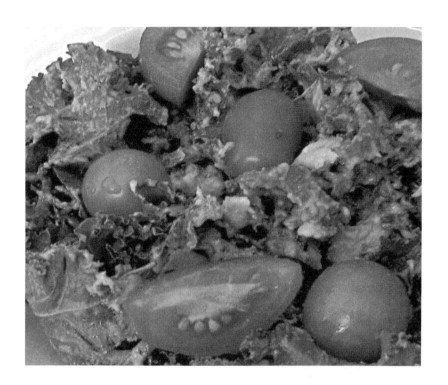

Ingredients:

Kale is a leafy vegetable that's excellent for your wellness! It is full of many vital vitamins.

One handful of organic kale stems removed 1/2 of an avocado☐

One tbsp. raw honey ☐

One tbsp. expeller pressed oil

1/4 cup natural (organic) apple-cider vinegar Pinch of sea-salt ☐

Squeeze half of a lemon

One carton natural cherry tomatoes, chopped in halves ☐

1/4 cup sunflower seeds

Directions:

Step 1

Rip kale into bits and put into a sizable salad bowl.

Step 2

Prep vinaigrette, mixing vinegar, olive oil, honey, salt, and orange juice in a mixer.

Step 3

Massages well until kale is softened then pour vinaigrette over it.

Step 4

Best with sunflower seeds and cherry tomatoes.

Delicious Warm Chicken and Potato

Salad with Peas and Mint

Serves 4-6

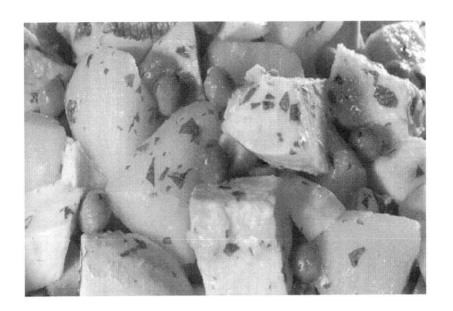

Ingredients:

9 - 12 new carrots peeled or scoured and reduce in to pieces salt and
newly ground black pepper

2 tbsps. cider vinegar

1 1/2, cups frozen garden peas, thawed

One small ripe avocado

4 chicken breasts (cooked), about I pound. In weight, skinned and diced

2 tbsps. freshly cut mint

2 heads little lettuce

Fresh mint sprigs, to garnish

Dressing:

2 tablespoons raspberry or sherry vinegar

2 tablespoons Dijon mustard

1 tablespoon clear honey

¼ cup sunflower oil

¼ cup extra-virgin olive oil

Directions:

Step 1

Prepare the potatoes in lightly salted cooking water for a fifteen minutes, or until just soft: don't overcook, Wash under running water to cool down a little, after that strain and turn into a sizable dish. Spread using the cider vinegar and toss lightly.

Step 2

Run the peas under warm water to add to the potatoes, pat dry with absorbent kitchen papers and ensure they are thawed

Step 3

Slice the avocado in two and get rid of the stone, Peel and chopped the avocado into dices and add the peas and potatoes, add the chicken and mix together gently,

Step 4

To make the dressing, place each of the ingredients in a screw-top container, with a little salt and pepper and shake well to blend: add a bit more oil if the flavor is sharp, Pour on the salad and toss lightly to coat. Spread in half the peppermint and mix softly.

Step 5

Divide the lettuce leaves and spread onto a big shallow serving plate, Spoon the salad at the top and mix with the rest of the mint. Garnish with mint sprigs and serve.

Pear Salad

Ingredients:

1 large bunch watercress or arugula

3 ripe pears

1 avocado

Dressing:

1/ 2 cup olive oil

3 tablespoons apple cider vinegar

2 teaspoon raw organic honey

1/ 4 teaspoon sea salt

1 tablespoon tomato paste

Directions:

Remove the stems from the watercress or arugula and wash well. Combine the dressing ingredients and set aside. Peel the pears and avocado, and slice them thinly.

Rinse the pear and avocados slices well, and arrange them over the greens on salad plates. Add the dressing and serve straightaway.

SOUP

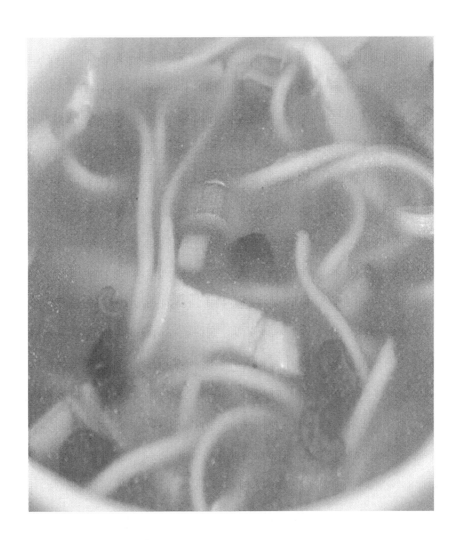

Amazing Oriental Noodle Hotpot

SERVES 8

COOKING TIME: 30 MINUTES

Serving noodles in an aromatic, spicy broth is a great method to ensure an appropriate portion size. The stock base for this soup is infused with garlic and ginger to give it a characteristic Asian flavor. Rounding out the broth and noodles are several key super foods: bean curd, carrots, cabbage and vinegar. In case you prefer, you can replace diced cooked chicken for the tofu.

Ingredients:

1.25 liters chicken or vegetable stock made without salt

3 slices (5mm thick) peeled fresh root ginger

2 garlic cloves, crushed

¼ teaspoon crushed dried chillies

2 teaspoons canola (rapeseed) oil

125g fresh shiitake mushrooms, stalks removed, wiped clean and sliced

½ medium head Chinese leaves or green cabbage, shredded

225g firm tofu, drained, patted dry and cut into 2.5cm cubes

3 medium carrots, grated

2 teaspoons reduced-salt soy sauce

2 teaspoons rice vinegar

1 teaspoon toasted sesame oil

125g whole meal linguine or spaghetti

2 medium spring onions, chopped

Directions:

- Bring a large saucepan of lightly salted water to the boil.

- Bring the stock to a simmer in another large saucepan. Add the ginger, garlic and chillies. Partly cover and simmer over a medium-low heat for 15 minutes to intensify the flavor. Strain the stock through a sieve into another large saucepan and discard the flavorings. Set the pan of stock aside.

- Heat the oil in a large non-stick frying pan over a medium-high heat. Add the sliced mushrooms and cook, stirring often, for 3-5 minutes or until tender. Add the Chinese leaves (or cabbage) and cook, stirring often, for a further 2-3 minutes or until almost tender.

- Add the mushrooms and Chinese leaves to the pan of infused stock. Simmer, partly covered over a medium-low heat for about 5 minutes or until the Chinese leaves are tender. Add the tofu and carrots and heat through. Stir in the soya sauce, vinegar and sesame oil.

- Meanwhile, cook the linguine (or spaghetti) in the boiling water for 6-9 minutes, or according to the packet instructions, until al dente. Drain the linguine and divide among four large soup bowls. Ladle the soup over the noodles and garnish each serving with the chopped spring onions.

PER SERVING: 110kcal, 6g protein, 15g carbohydrate, 3g fiber, 3.5 total fat, 3.5g saturated fat, 0mg cholesterol, 0.5g salt.

MAIN COURSES

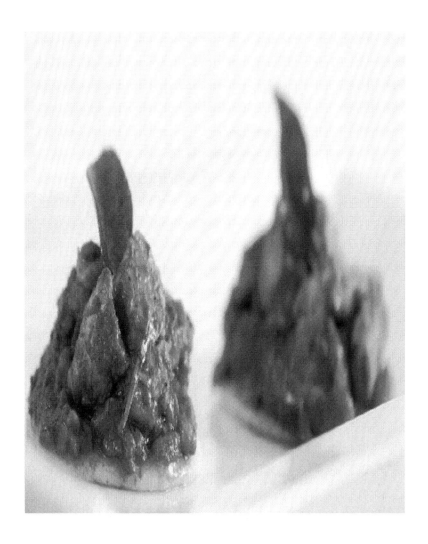

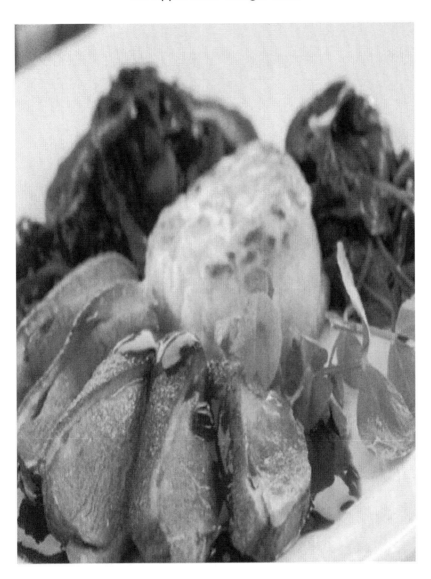

Rump Steak with Balsamic Sauce

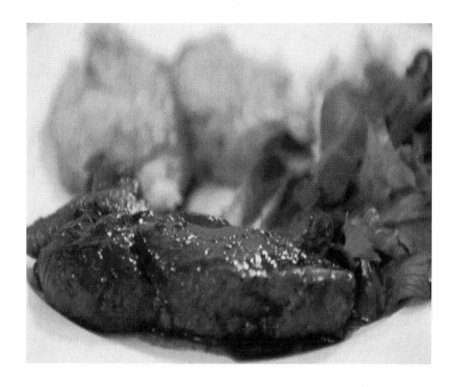

Serve 6

Marinating Time: 2 hours

Cooking Time: 12-14 Minutes

Rump steak has tons of flavor, and turn out to be soft and extremely succulent when marinated. It is simple to control portion sizes, because you slit the steak before serving. In this recipe, the marinade is changed into a sauce.

Ingredients:

85ml port wine or fresh orange juice

1 tbsp. Worcestershire sauce

4 tbsps. balsamic vinegar

1 tbsp. sliced thyme or one tbsp. dried thyme

Fresh black pepper to flavor

700g rump steak, cut

2 tbsps. finely chopped shallot

1 tbsp. olive oil

Small button of unsalted butter (about 10g)

Directions:

Step 1

In a little dish, whisk together the juice from the orange (or port), salt and pepper, sauce, vinegar, Worcestershire, thyme and garlic. Put the meat in a short glass dish, pour over the orange liquid mixture and turn to coat. Cover and leave to marinate in the fridge for two hours or around eight hours, rotating a few times.

Step 2

Empty the marinade into a smaller saucepan as soon as you remove the steak. Add the shallot and put aside. Warm a ridged griddle pan (or perhaps a large frying pan). Brush with the oil, then add the steak and cook over a heat for six to seven minutes on each side (depending on the depth of the steak). Cook for longer, should you prefer your meat well done. Transfer to a chopping board and allow to rest for five minutes.

Step 3

In the meantime, over a medium to high heat bring the marinade to the boil and cook for three to five minutes or until lowered to about 5 tablespoons.

Step 4

Cut the steak in thin slices across the grain. Include any collected juices from the chopping board over the dressing and offer the dressing with the meat. Any leftover steak may be kept, covered, in the fridge for up to two days.

PER SERVING: 183kcal, 26g protein, 4.5g carbohydrate, 0g fiber, 7g total fat, 3g saturated fat, 7mg cholesterol, 0.6g salt.

Tasty Creamy Turkey and Tomato Pasta

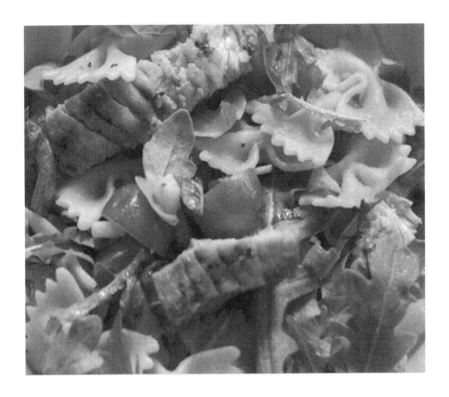

Serve 4

Ingredients:

2 garlic cloves, peeled and chopped

1 teaspoon turkey breasts, cut into bite-sized pieces

1 ¼ 1b cherry tomatoes, on the vine

4 teaspoons neatly cut basil

4 teaspoons olive oil

4 teaspoons balsamic vinegar

salt and ground black pepper

12 oz. tagliatelle

¾ crème fraiche

shaved Parmesan cheese, to garnish

Directions:

Step 1

Preheat the oven to Gas Mark 5 or 6, Heat 2 tablespoons of olive oil in a big frying pan, Add the turkey and cook for five minutes, turning occasionally.

Transfer to a roasting container and include the rest of the olive oil, balsamic vinegar, garlic and the vine tomatoes, Stir well and season to taste with salt and pepper, Cook in the preheated oven for 30 minutes, or until the turkey is soft, turning the tomatoes and turkey once.

Step 2

At the same time, bring a big pan, of lightly salted water to a boil. Add the pasta. Drain, return to the pan and keep warm. Stir the basil and seasoning into the crème fraiche.

Step 3

Take out the roasting container from the oven and dispose the vines, Stir the crème fraiche and basil mix into the turkey and tomato mixture then return to the oven for another one to two minutes.

Step 4

Stir the turkey and tomato mixture into the pasta and shake gently together, transfer into a warm serving dish. Garnish with Parmesan cheese shavings and serve right away.

Roasted Lamb with Rosemary and Garlic

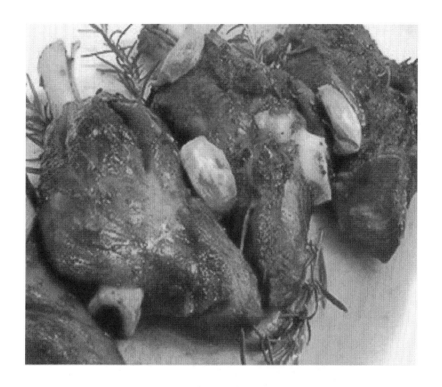

Serve 6

Ingredients:

3 1/2 1b leg of lamb

few sprigs of clean rosemary

8 garlic cloves, (peeled)

4 pieces pancetta

6 medium potatoes

sprigs of fresh rosemary, to garnish

salt and ground black pepper

4 tablespoons red-wine vinegar

4 tablespoon olive oil

One large onion

freshly cooked ratatouille, to serve

Directions:

Step 1

In the meantime preheat the oven to Gas Mark 5 or 6, about fifteen minutes before placing the roasting the lamb. Clean the lamb using a damp material, and then put the lamb in a sizable roasting tin.

Using a sharp knife, make small and deep incisions in the meat, chop two to three cloves of garlic into little slivers, after that add a couple rosemary sprigs to the leg of lamb. Add pepper and salt to taste then cover the leg of lamb with the small pieces of pancetta.

Step 2

Sprinkle one tablespoon olive oil then put a couple more rosemary sprigs over the leg of lamb. Roast for half an hour and then drizzle over the vinegar.

Step 3

Peel the onion and cut into thick wedges then thickly slice the rest of the garlic. In the meantime, peel the potatoes and cut into large dice. Arrange round the lamb.

Pour the rest of the olive oil over the potatoes, then reduce the oven temperature to Gas Mark 4 and roast for an additional one hour, or until the lamb is soft. Garnish with fresh sprigs of rosemary and serve immediately with the roast potatoes and ratatouille.

SIDE DISHES

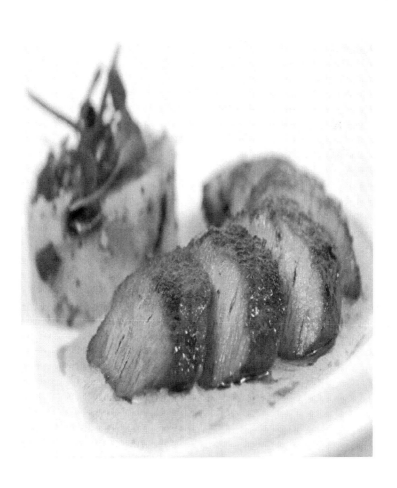

Sautéed Brussels Sprouts With

Red Pepper and Caraway Seeds

Serve 4

Cooking Time: 12 Minutes

This sturdy vegetable is loaded with super benefits. Sautéed with red pepper, sprouts make a superb side dish to go along with lean meat for an easy midweek supper.

Ingredients:

300 grams Brussels sprouts, cut and cored

2 teaspoons canola (rapeseed) oil

1 medium onion, sliced

1 medium red pepper, deseeded and cut into 5cm lengthy slivers

1 1/2 teaspoons caraway seeds

125ml vegetable or chicken stock made without salt

3 tablespoons cider vinegar

1/4 teaspoon salt, or to flavor

Ground black pepper to flavor

Directions:

Step 1

Quarter the Brussels sprouts with a razor-sharp blade knife, or shred them in a food processor equipped with the disk.

Step 2

Heat the oil in a sizable non-stick baking pan over a moderate to high heat. Add the red pepper and onion and cook, stirring often, for 3-4 minutes or until tender.

Step 3

Include the Brussels sprouts and sauté them, stirring, for two minutes. Put in the stock. Cover the pot and cook for an additional two to three minutes or until the sprouts are soft but still have some chew to it. Stir in the salt and pepper and cider vinegar and serve hot.

PER SERVING: 66kcal, 3.3g protein, 7.5g carbohydrate, 4g fiber, 2.7g total fat, 0.5g saturated fat, 0mg cholesterol, 0.3g salt.

Sautéed Spinach with Ginger and Soy Sauce

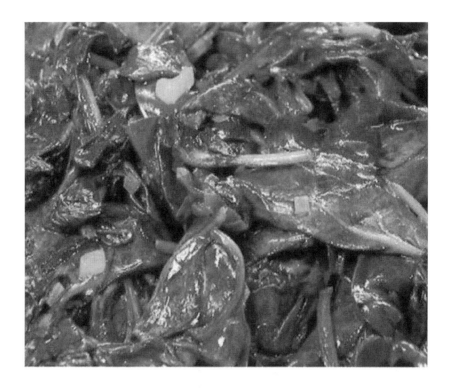

Serve 2

Cooking Time: 5-8 Minutes

This one has an oriental twist and uses aromatic sesame oil, which is low in saturated fat.

Ingredients:

300g fresh spinach, large stalks trimmed off and leaves thoroughly washed

1 tablespoon reduced-salt soy sauce

2 teaspoons rice vinegar

1 teaspoon toasted sesame oil

½ teaspoon soft brown sugar

2 teaspoons canola (rapeseed) oil

1 garlic clove, finely chopped

1 ½ teaspoons finely chopped fresh root ginger

Pinch of crushed dried chillies

1 tablespoon sesame seeds, toasted

Directions:

Step 1

Sauté the spinach (with just the water clinging to the leaves after washing) in a large, wide pan over a medium-high heat for 3-5 minutes or until wilted. Drain, rinse with cold water and press out excess moisture.

Step 2

Mix the soya sauce vinegar, sesame oil and sugar together in a small bowl. Heat the oil in a large non-stick frying pan over a medium- high heat.

Add the garlic, ginger and chillies, and stir-fry for about 10 seconds or until fragrant but not browned.

Add the spinach and cook, stirring often, for 2-3 minutes or until heated through. Stir in the soy sauce mixture and toss to coat well. Sprinkle with the sesame seeds and serve.

PER SERVING: 129kcal, 6g protein, 5g carbohydrate, 4g fiber, 10g total fat, 1.5g saturated fat, 0mg cholesterol, 1.32g salt.

Spinach with Pine Nuts and Currants

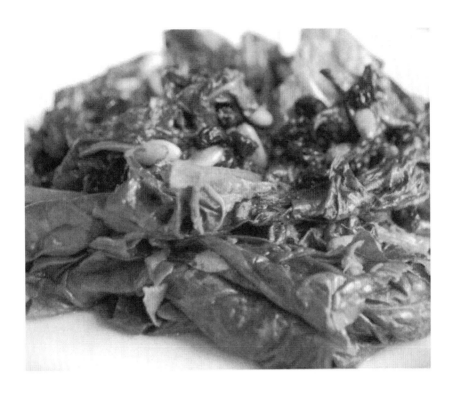

Serve 4

Cooking Time: 5-8 Minutes

You can include a side-dish of Super spinach in your weekly menu plan, because frozen spinach works flawlessly in this version of a traditional Spanish recipe, even though you haven't had time to buy fresh vegetables.

Use the frozen chopped spinach that's packed loose, rather than spinach frozen in a block, as it is much easier to sauté.

Ingredients:

50g currants or coarsely sliced raisins

500g frozen cut green spinach

35g pine nuts

2 teaspoons pure olive oil

1 medium onion carefully cut

1/2 teaspoon salt, or to flavor

1 tablespoon balsamic vinegar

1 garlic clove, finely chopped

Ground black pepper to taste

Directions:

Step 1

Place the raisins or currants in a little dish and put enough boiling water to cover. Leave to plump up for five to ten minutes. Drain, saving the soaking liquid.

Step 2

Heat the oil in a large non-stick frying pan on a medium-low heat. Add the pine nuts and cook, stirring, for one to two minutes or till light golden brown. Transfer the pine nuts into a small pan and set aside.

Step 3

Add the garlic and onion to the pan. Cook, stirring, for two to three minutes or until softened and light golden. Now add the frozen kale and 2 tbsps. of the reserved soaking liquid.

Increase the heat to medium high and cook, stirring, for three to five minutes or until the spinach is entirely thawed and piping hot. Stir in the pine nuts and currants. Season with the vinegar, salt and pepper, and serve.

PER SERVING: 152kcal, 5g protein, 13g carbohydrate, 3.4g fiber, 8.6g total fat, 0.7g saturated fat, 0mg cholesterol, 0.9g salt.

DESSERTS

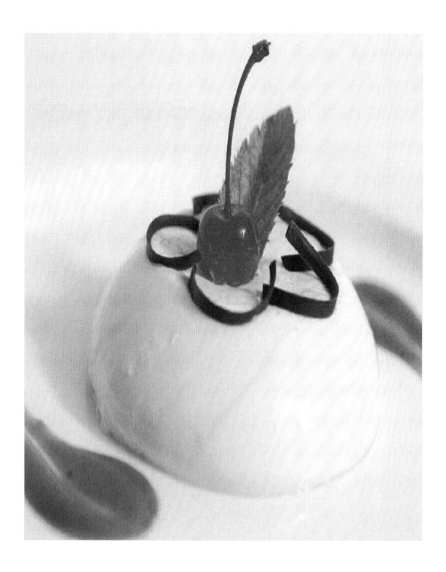

Fruity Meringue Crush

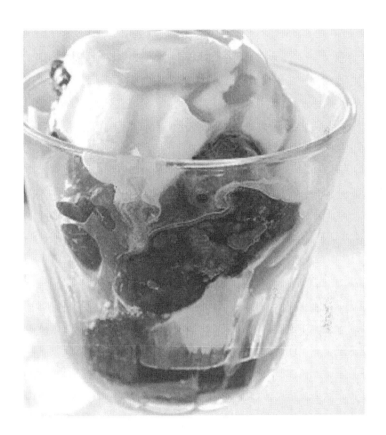

Ingredients:

4 scoops of Vanilla Snow Cream (100g/200ml)

4 meringues

100g raspberries

4 half strawberries

1 tbsp. balsamic vinegar

1 tbsp. icing sugar

100g strawberries, hulled and diced

4 sprigs of mint

Directions:

Step 1

Combine the balsamic vinegar, raspberries, strawberries and frosting sugar together in a little dish.

Step 2

Crush the meringues gentle in a big dish and combine with all the Vanilla Ice Cream.

Step 3

Fold the blended berries lightly into the ice cream mixture and meringue.

Step 4

Divide the mix between 4 serving glasses and then garnish each with half a strawberry and a sprig of mint. Serve straight away.

Balsamic Flavored Strawberries

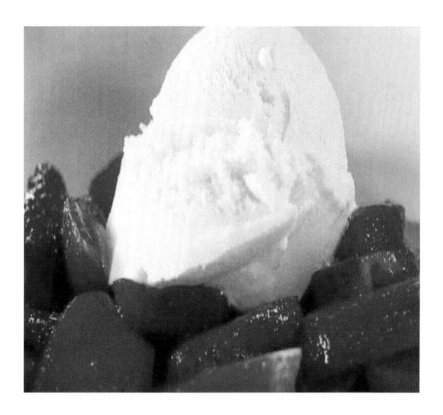

Ingredients:

9 cups strawberries of freshly thick sliced

2 tbsps. sugar

5 tbsps. balsamic vinegar

2 pts. vanilla ice cream

1/4 tbsp. ground black pepper

grated lemon zest (Freshly)

Directions

Step 1

Thirty minutes before serving, Mix the pepper, balsamic vinegar, strawberries, and sugar in a dish. Put aside at room-temperature.

Step 2

Place a portion of the berries in a dish with a scoop of ice-cream on top then dust with a little orange zest.

ABOUT THE AUTHOR

Even though sarcasm is commonly her tone, she counts on her friends to understand that underneath it is a gentle soul. She lives in sunny Florida, the city of her birth. Elena had a long career as a nutritionist.

As a young adult she developed her acid free approach of treating and curing psoriasis. She is married to a fantastic man who has a heart of gold. She has one son and two daughters. Elena spends her time skiing, jogging and hiking with her dog harry.

IN CLOSING. . . . .

So there you've got it. Was that enjoyable, interesting and insightful? I sincerely hope so. As I mentioned at the beginning of this book, I had the opportunity to learn all of the wisdom through my own personal experiences with cider vinegar and I found it enjoyable.

Whether your interest is really in food that's both healthy and delicious, or in finding out if it works for you personally like a treatment, you cannot afford to be without vinegar.

DEAR READER!

May you be on your way to a happier, more relaxed, less stressful and healthier life!

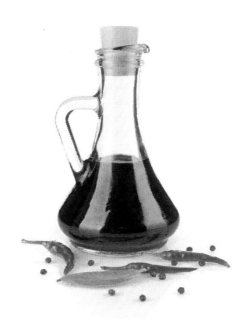